The SCIENCE Report on Heart Research

COMBATING THE #1 KILLER

The SCIENCE Report on Heart Research

Jean L. Marx and Gina Bari Kolata

With a Preface by Jeremiah Stamler, M.D.

American Association for the Advancement of Science

Library of Congress Cataloging in Publication Data

Marx, Jean L.
  Combating the #1 killer: the SCIENCE report on heart
research.

  Bibliography: p.
  Includes index.
  1. Heart — Diseases — Research I. Kolata, Gina Bari, joint
author. II. Science. III. Title.
RC681.M385   616.1'2   78-3626
ISBN 0-87168-219-2   ,
ISBN 0-87168-235-4 pbk.

AAAS Publication 78-3

Part of the material in this book originally appeared as a series in the
Research News section of SCIENCE, the Journal of the American
Association for the Advancement of Science. The authors are members of
the Research News staff of SCIENCE.

Printed in the United States of America

Contents

$17.00

List of Illustrations

Acknowledgements

The authors would like to thank their colleagues at *Science* for their support and encouragement, Fanny Groom for her typing and clerical assistance, and the many scientists and physicians who generously offered their time and guidance while we were researching and writing this book. The authors especially acknowledge the many helpful suggestions and criticisms of William Kolata.

—J.L.M. and G.B.K.

Preface

Heart attack is the great plague — the mass epidemic — of modern times in economically developed countries. Its annual toll in sickness, disability, and death is in the millions in the United States alone, and a sizable proportion of the victims are young and middle-aged adults.

The pathologic process underlying heart attack is advanced atherosclerosis of the coronary arteries. And severe atherosclerosis also occurs frequently in major arteries supplying the brain, trunk, and lower extremities, with consequent cerebrovascular disease (stroke), arterial aneurysm, gangrene, and other catastrophic illness.

Given the extent and seriousness of this problem — atherosclerotic disease (not cancer) is the Number One crippler and killer in the United States — research on atherosclerotic disease appropriately became a major focus of biomedical investigators after World War II. In the escalating and by now extensive efforts to elucidate the nature, etiology, pathogenesis, and means of preventing and controlling this disease, every approach available to biomedical science has been used: epidemiology, clinical and pathologic investigation, and animal experimentation. A tremendous amount of productive work has been done and much has been learned. The specific research reports number in the tens of thousands, the reviews and monographs in the hundreds. For scientists in the field, keeping up with the literature in even one area, that is, reading, assimilating, and digesting it, plus systematically summarizing and evaluating it for publication, has become a major, often forbidding task, as this writer has learned painfully from long experience!

Therefore, this book by Jean L. Marx and Gina Bari Kolata, reporters of the biomedical scene for *Science,* is an outstanding accomplishment. They have put together an important, up-to-date overview of the status of research on atherosclerosis and the major adult cardiovascular diseases.

This book is valuable precisely because its main focus is on key research in progress, on the ever-shifting frontier between the known and the unknown. A difficult undertaking of this kind on the major aspects of a big problem is bound to contain formulations that researchers deeply involved in the work will question, and they will almost inevitably also be concerned about "significant" omissions. Here the aphorism of Hippocrates continues to be timely: "Life is short, and the art long," both for science writers and science practitioners! The point, particularly for all who are immersed in the work, is to avoid losing the forest for the trees. Ms. Marx and Ms. Kolata have produced a book replete with information and insight for investigators in the field, scientists generally, makers of public policy, and the public at large.

Perhaps the most exciting aspect of the cardiovascular disease scene at this moment is the steady decline in mortality rates in the United States since 1968, noted by the authors in Chapter 1. For young and middle-aged adults, the decrease in heart attack death rates was by 1975 in excess of 20 percent, and the drop in mortality rates due to stroke was even greater. If the 1968 death rates had prevailed in 1975, over 100,000 additional persons would have died from heart attack and stroke in that single year of latest record. This is the measure of the lives saved. As a consequence, mortality from all causes, the "bottom line," is also down significantly. Life expectancy for adult Americans, men and women, white and black, is longer than ever before recorded.

True, U.S. death rates from the atherosclerotic diseases still are among the highest in the world. But the decrease in the death rate from cardiovascular diseases between 1968 and 1975 shows that this onslaught, like epidemics that were ended in previous eras, is neither inevitable nor immutable. We are learning more about how atherosclerotic disease can be prevented and controlled.

For 20 years, expert committees established by the American Heart Association, the Inter-Society Commission for Heart Disease Resources, the White House Conference on Nutrition, and the National Heart, Lung, and Blood Institute have been bringing to the health professions, the custodians of public policy, and the public the growing bodies of research data indicating that the epidemic of adult cardiovascular diseases is a result of life-styles and of major risk factors related to life-styles. They have been urging improved patterns of eating, smoking, and exercise in order to prevent and control this epidemic. Evidence is available that the American people have been responding to these recommendations, as well as to advice about the importance of effective, long-term treatment of established high blood pressure. And it is entirely possible that the recent sizable declines in the mortality rates attributable to cardiovascular diseases are at least in part byproducts of these changes, as well as of the application of new knowledge about the acute and long-term medical treatment of those already ill from atherosclerotic diseases.

This book, by bringing to its readers a contemporary account of research progress on this major problem, should serve to extend understanding of the importance of the continuing investigative effort. It is also important that its findings be brought to bear promptly and effectively in the treatment of the sick — but above all — in expanding and intensifying the strategically decisive preventive effort.

JEREMIAH STAMLER, M.D.

Epidemiology

1

CARDIOVASCULAR DISEASE
Its Forms and Its Victims

Cardiovascular diseases—diseases of the heart and blood vessels—are the leading cause of death in this country. They afflict more than 29 million people and are responsible for about 1 million deaths per year in the United States alone (Figure 1). Half of all deaths in this country can be attributed to cardiovascular diseases. Although the incidence of these diseases increases with age, they are not limited to the elderly; one-fourth of all heart attack deaths occur before the age of 65. Even children are vulnerable to some forms of heart disease, especially those caused by birth defects and rheumatic fever.

Not only do the cardiovascular diseases inflict a high cost in human suffering (Figures 2 and 3), but in addition, their economic cost is high. The American Heart Association (AHA) estimates that the total economic cost of these diseases in 1978 will be in excess of $28 billion (Figure 4). Medical expenses account for $20 billion of this sum, and the other $8 billion is attributed to lost output due to disability.

Nevertheless, government funding of research into the causes and treatment of diseases of the heart and blood vessels has lagged significantly behind that of cancer research. Passage by Congress of the Heart, Lung, and Blood Act of 1972 did improve the situation, however. The budget of the National Heart, Lung, and Blood Institute (NHLBI) has increased from $233 million for fiscal year (FY) 1972 to $397 million for FY 1977. In addition, the AHA spent almost $20 million for research in 1977. (For comparison, the total

3

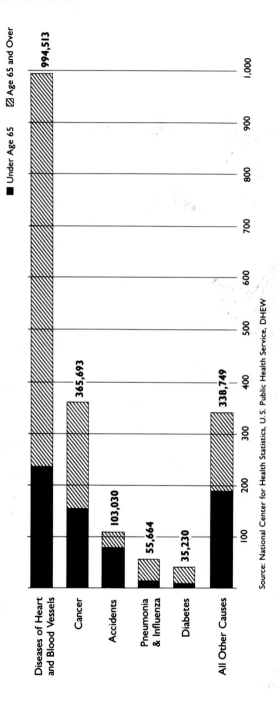

Figure 1. The leading causes of death in the United States in 1975. Numbers of deaths are shown at the bottom of the columns in thousands. [© Reprinted with the permission of the American Heart Association]

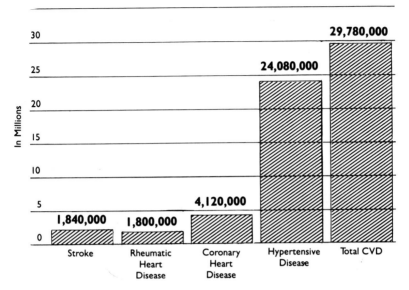

Figure 2. Estimated prevalance of the major cardiovascular diseases (CVD) in the United States in 1975. The sum of the individual estimates exceeds 29,780,000 since many persons have more than one cardiovascular disorder. [© Reprinted with the permission of the American Heart Association]

budget of the National Cancer Institute for FY 1977 was almost $816 million.)

The public might justifiably ask, what does this money buy? This book examines some of the recent developments in research on cardiovascular diseases, with special emphasis on progress being made in efforts to understand the biological mechanisms underlying the diseases. The research is providing the kind of information needed to prevent or cure a disease – not just to control its symptoms. Clinical advances in treating hypertension and abnormal heart rhythms, in limiting the damage to heart muscle caused by heart attacks, and in detecting and measuring the extent of heart disease will also be considered. Although the money spent for research has not yet eliminated cardiovascular disease as the leading cause of death, the research is laying the foundation that may one day permit the attainment of that goal.

Much of the research has been directed toward uncovering the causes of heart attacks and strokes. These are the most spectacular – and lethal – manifestations of cardiovascular disease. Together they claim nearly 840,000 victims every year (Figure 3). Although heart

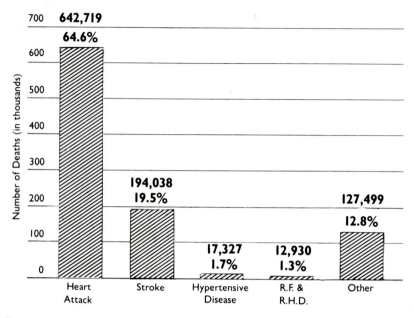

Figure 3. Deaths due to the major cardiovascular disorders in the United States in 1975. Rheumatic fever and rheumatic heart disease are abbreviated as R.F. and R.H.D., respectively. Source: National Center for Health Statistics, USPHS, DHEW. [© Reprinted with the permission of the American Heart Association]

attacks and strokes appear to occur suddenly, they are actually the result of a subtle, long-term deterioration of the circulatory system.

A heart attack is the result of blockage of one or more of the three coronary arteries that normally supply blood to the heart muscle. This blockage cuts off the supply of oxygen and other nutrients to a portion of the heart muscle (myocardium). The area receiving insufficient blood flow is said to be "ischemic." Some, although not necessarily all, of the ischemic tissue eventually dies, and the dead segment is called an "infarct." Myocardial infarct, coronary occlusion, and coronary thrombosis (blood clot) are all synonyms for heart attack.

If the damage is so extensive that the heart cannot function, the individual dies. But even less severe damage may disrupt the electrical impulses that originate in the heart's internal pacemaker and regulate the heartbeat. This disruption will produce abnormal heart rhythms (cardiac arrhythmias). Certain of these are very dangerous because they may result in ventricular fibrillation; that

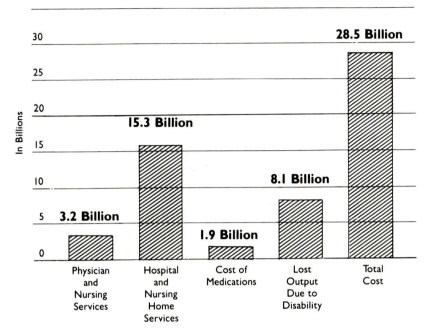

Figure 4. The estimated economic cost of cardiovascular disease in the United States in 1978. [© Reprinted with the permission of the American Heart Association]

is, the rapid, uncoordinated contraction of the large chambers of the heart. Death may occur within minutes unless the normal heart rhythm is restored. Ventricular fibrillation can also result from heart injuries or abnormalities other than blockage of the coronary arteries.

Sometimes heart attacks are caused by the trapping in the coronary arteries of a blood clot formed elsewhere in the body; usually, however, blockage of the arteries is the result of the formation of atherosclerotic plaques. The plaques develop gradually over a period of many years. They contain an accumulation of smooth muscle cells from the arterial wall; lipids, especially cholesterol; and calcium. (Atherosclerosis refers specifically to the development of these plaques in the arteries. Arteriosclerosis is a general term for the condition in which the arteries thicken, harden and lose their elasticity. Atherosclerosis is one type of arteriosclerosis.)

Atherosclerotic plaques serve as initiation sites for the formation of blood clots that can block the arteries. In addition, the plaques themselves may build up to the point where they partially block the coronary arteries. When this happens, the heart muscle gets enough oxygen when the individual is at rest but not during exertion. Transient pain results, a condition called angina pectoris. The conditions characterized by inadequate supply of oxygen to the heart are collectively called coronary heart (or artery) disease. More than 4 million persons in the United States have a history of heart attack or angina pectoris*.

Atherosclerosis can affect and block any artery. If the lesions form in the arteries of the leg, for example, blood flow to the extremity may be cut off, causing numbness, pain, and ultimately gangrene if not treated. If the arteries blocked by atherosclerotic plaques are in the brain, stroke may result and a portion of the brain will be damaged. Alternatively, stroke may be caused when one of the blood vessels in the brain bursts. This kind of stroke is most likely to occur in persons who have uncontrolled high blood pressure, especially if they also have atherosclerosis. About 1.8 million persons in this country have suffered strokes, which cause about 200,000 deaths per year.

High blood pressure, also called hypertension, is a major risk factor, not just for stroke but also for heart attack and atherosclerosis. Hypertension does not produce overt symptoms unless it is severe or has been untreated for a long time. But it puts a strain on the heart, which is forced to work harder in order to move the blood against higher than normal pressures. An enlarged heart is one result of high blood pressure. Hypertension may also contribute to the development of atherosclerosis by damaging arterial walls. Kidney failure is another consequence of prolonged, elevated blood pressure. More than 24 million persons are estimated to have high blood pressure — and only about 30 percent of them have it adequately controlled even though it is easy to detect and effective therapies are available.

Rheumatic heart disease usually afflicts children between the ages of 5 and 15. It often begins with a severe throat infection caused by streptococcal bacteria ("strep throat"). A small percentage of infected persons make antibodies against the bacteria that attack and damage the heart valves and muscle with the result that blood can no longer be effectively pumped. Mortality from rheumatic fever

---

* The figures cited in this chapter are taken from the 1978 edition of the *Heart Facts* pamphlet published by the American Heart Association (7320 Greenville Avenue, Dallas, Texas 75231).

has decreased because antibiotics can control strep infections, and diseased valves can be surgically repaired. But approximately 13,000 people in this country still die every year as a result of rheumatic heart disease.

Congenital defects also contribute to the toll from cardiovascular disease. About 25,000 infants are born every year in the United States with defects of the heart or major blood vessels. Some of these are the result of rubella infection of the mother during the first 3 months of pregnancy. Vaccination programs have contributed to a decrease in the number of these defects. Other defects are of unknown origin, but many can now be corrected surgically.

Still another cardiovascular disease, congestive heart failure, occurs when the heart has been weakened, whether by high blood pressure, heart attack, rheumatic heart disease, or birth defects, and pumps well below its normal capacity. Loss of pumping power by the heart results in fluid accumulation in the abdomen, legs, and lungs, making breathing difficult. Congestive heart failure can be effectively treated with drugs.

2

EPIDEMIOLOGY OF HEART DISEASE
Search for Causes

Medical scientists would like very much to know what causes cardiovascular diseases in the hope that this knowledge would permit prevention of the diseases and a large reduction in the death rate. The causes, if any simple ones exist, have eluded investigators despite the expenditures of large amounts of time and money. However, several factors that appear to contribute to the development of cardiovascular diseases have been identified. The evidence comes from the results of three types of research: epidemiological, biochemical, and clinical. This chapter will concentrate on the epidemiological studies; others will discuss some of the biochemical and clinical evidence concerning the etiology of heart disease.

Epidemiology often parallels the other types of research by providing indications of what conditions are associated with or predispose people to develop cardiovascular diseases. Biochemical and clinical methods can then be used to investigate the mechanisms by which the conditions cause the diseases and to determine whether modifying the conditions can prevent the diseases.

Since World War II, epidemiologists have studied populations all over the world to see whether the incidence of cardiovascular diseases varies among different populations. They found that the incidence does vary and is related to several risk factors, particularly cigarette smoking, high blood pressure, and high concentrations of serum cholesterol (Figures 5 and 6, pp. 12–14).

Observations of long-term trends in mortality in general and in mortality due to cardiovascular diseases in particular may also shed light on the possible causes of these diseases. Such observations have recently revealed an encouraging fact: the death rate from cardiovascular diseases in the United States has declined markedly during the past several years.

In 1975, according to investigators at the National Center for Health Statistics, 979,180 people in the United States died of the major cardiovascular diseases. This is the first year since 1967 that the number of such deaths was less than 1 million. The conditions included as major cardiovascular diseases by the center are hypertension and hypertensive heart disease; coronary heart disease, including heart attacks and angina pectoris; stroke; chronic diseases of the heart muscle or membranes; heart failure and shock; and arteriosclerosis. Congenital heart defects and diseases of the veins, such as phlebitis, were not included.

The death rates, calculated for each age group or adjusted to compensate for the changing age distribution of the population, for all the categories of major cardiovascular disease have been dropping since 1968. Cardiologists are especially gratified by the decrease in the death rate from coronary heart disease, which killed approximately 640,000 people in 1975 and which is the biggest contributer to the overall cardiovascular death rate. Between 1970 and 1975, the decrease was 13 percent, saving about 15,000 lives per year. This is an apparent reversal of a trend that began before 1940. Between 1940 and 1960 the mortality rate from coronary heart disease increased steadily. It plateaued between 1960 and 1967 and then began decreasing.

Epidemiologists would like to see the trend continue for a few more years in order to be sure it is not a statistical quirk. Most believe the trend is real, but no one has a sure explanation for it.

Since high blood pressure, cigarette smoking, and high concentrations of serum cholesterol are thought to predispose people to develop heart disease, investigators are asking whether decreases in the frequency of these traits in the U.S. population may have contributed to the decrease in mortality from cardiovascular diseases. So far, the evidence is suggestive but inconclusive.

Hypertension can be treated with drugs, and there is evidence that adequate control of this condition can decrease the risk of developing cardiovascular diseases. The death rate from hypertension itself dropped 28 percent from 1970 to 1975. But the contribution

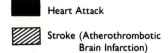

■ Heart Attack

▨ Stroke (Atherothrombotic
Brain Infarction)

a. Cigarette Smoking

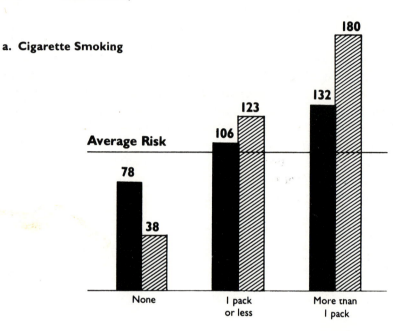

Average Risk

	None	I pack or less	More than I pack
Heart Attack	78	106	132
Stroke	38	123	180

b. Cholesterol

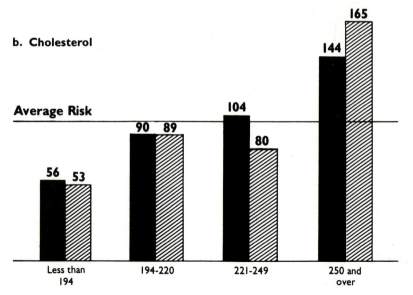

Average Risk

	Less than 194	194-220	221-249	250 and over
Heart Attack	56	90	104	144
Stroke	53	89	80	165

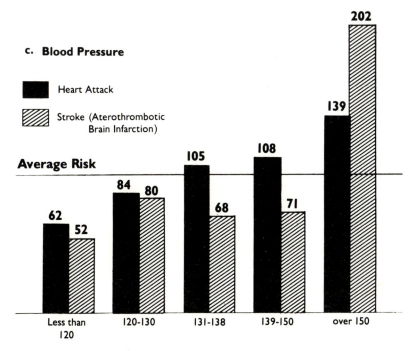

Figure 5.   The risk factors for heart attack and stroke. The graphs show the extent to which cigarette smoking (a), elevated blood cholesterol concentrations (b), and high blood pressure (c) increase the risk of having a heart attack or stroke. The risks increase as the number of cigarettes smoked per day, cholesterol concentrations, and blood pressures increase. The figures listed below the bars in (b) are blood cholesterol concentrations expressed as milligrams per 100 milliliters of blood. In (c), the figures below the bars represent systolic blood pressures. [Source: Reprinted with the permission of the Framingham, Mass., Heart Study]

of drug treatment to the decrease in mortality cannot be evaluated yet. One anomaly is that the downward trend in the rates began before the drugs became widely available, according to Tavia Gordon and Thomas Thom of the Biometrics Research Branch of the National Heart, Lung, and Blood Institute (NHLBI).

Nevertheless, recent survey data compiled by the National High Blood Pressure Education Program of the NHLBI indicate that between 1971 and 1974 there was a significant increase in the percentage of cases of hypertension that were disgnosed. Moreover, it appears that a higher percentage of persons who are aware of their high blood pressure have their condition under control than before 1971. One problem with this analysis is that the population surveyed in 1974 may not be comparable to that surveyed previously. Nonetheless, many investigators think that better control of hypertension may be contributing to the downward trend in cardiovascular mortality.

Results of studies carried out by the American Cancer Society (ACS) indicate that the recent decrease in cigarette smoking and the shift to low-tar, low-nicotine cigarettes may have contributed to the

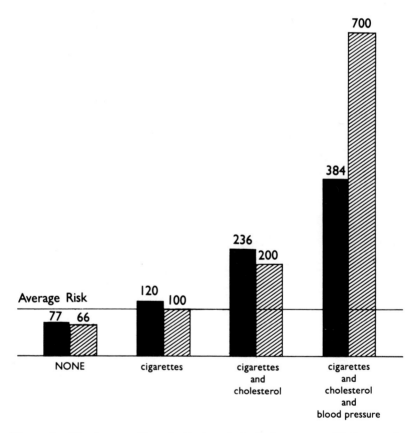

Figure 6. The danger of heart attack and stroke increases with the number of risk factors present. The example given is for a 45-year-old man; the high blood cholesterol concentration is 310 milligrams per 100 milliliters, and the elevated blood pressure (systolic) is 180. [Source: Reprinted with the permission of the Framingham, Mass., Heart Study]

decline in mortality from cardiovascular diseases. Persons taking part in these studies who smoked cigarettes low in tar and nicotine had lower death rates from both lung cancer and coronary heart disease than participants who smoked comparable numbers of high-tar, high-nicotine cigarettes. Nonsmokers, however, still fared much better than smokers of even the low-tar cigarettes. Robert Levy, director of the NHLBI, points out that the carbon monoxide present in cigarette smoke may contribute to the development of heart attacks but not of lung cancer so that a cigarette "safe" for the lung may not necessarily be "safe" for the heart.

Despite the results of the ACS studies, the effects of changing smoking habits on the mortality rates for cardiovascular diseases have not yet been determined. For example, more men than women have stopped smoking, but Gordon and Thom say that both sexes have experienced equal decreases in mortality from these diseases. Sorting out the effects of cigarette smoking from those of other risk factors whose prevalence differs between the two sexes will not be easy.

The role of changes in diet is especially complex. Jeremiah Stamler of Northwestern University Medical School says that people in this country have decreased their consumption of some foods with high cholesterol and saturated fat content (including eggs, whole milk, and butter) but have increased their consumption of other foods, beef in particular. Consequently, it is difficult to assess the net effect of these changes on the cholesterol and fat content of diets, and whether such changes have affected mortality from heart disease.

Besides looking for evidence that Americans may have changed their living habits, investigators have asked whether other factors may have affected mortality rates from cardiovascular diseases. One possibility, which improves the likelihood that people who suffer heart attacks will survive, is better medical care. This effect would be magnified by the widespread availability of coronary care units, specially trained ambulance crews, pacemakers to regulate the heart beat, and cardiopulmonary resuscitation techniques. But, as Stamler points out, the impact of coronary care units is necessarily limited by the fact that 70 percent of heart attack victims die before they reach the hospital.

During the last few years, there has been a dramatic increase in the number of coronary bypass operations. Richard Ross of the Johns

Hopkins University Medical School estimates that about 65,000 patients per year now undergo this procedure, in which diseased and blocked coronary arteries are replaced with healthy blood vessels taken from another part of the body. Although cardiologists agree that the operation can relieve the symptoms of severe, intractable coronary heart disease, no one knows whether it improves long-term survival rates. Stamler says that it is not now possible to determine whether the operation has had any impact on heart disease mortality rates.

Gordon and Thom suggest that the trend in coronary heart disease mortality rates may not result from voluntary actions of the American people. They point out that there has been a general decrease in the death rates from virtually all causes, with only a few exceptions such as cancer, accidents, and violence. Respiratory infections, such as influenza and pneumonia, often contribute to the deaths of people weakened by other diseases, including those of the circulatory system. Because the influenza epidemics since 1968 have killed comparatively few people, Gordon and Thom think that the decrease in the death rate from coronary disease may result in part from the freedom from the stress of influenza.

The difficulties faced by epidemiologists in explaining trends in mortality rates from cardiovascular diseases are typical of the problems that occur in the statistical study of all phases of these diseases. Results both from prospective studies, in which large groups of people are followed for years to see what characterizes those who develop cardiovascular diseases, and from retrospective comparisons of incidences of cardiovascular diseases among different populations, may sometimes vary from study to study in unexpected ways.

Gordon says that he and other epidemiologists tend not to believe any result until it has been repeated in several well-designed studies. Diabetes, high concentrations of serum cholesterol, cigarette smoking, and high blood pressure are correlated with risks of developing cardiovascular diseases in nearly all published studies. These conditions are thus accepted as risk factors by most investigators, even though a few studies may appear to exonerate one or another of them. Other factors, however, such as lack of exercise, which have been implicated as risk factors in a few studies, are not accepted as proven independent risk factors by the vast majority of epidemiologists because most investigators have not found a consistent relationship between these factors and cardiovascular disease.

In an ideal situation, the presence of a certain condition would virtually guarantee that a person will develop cardiovascular disease. The problem is that cardiovascular diseases seem to have so many causes that the ideal situation never occurs. Demonstrating cause and effect relationships is further complicated by the long latent period before cardiovascular disease becomes evident. Levy estimates that two to five decades can elapse before conditions that cause these diseases exhibit their effects.

To further complicate matters, it has been impossible to carry out an unbiased epidemiological study. For example, lack of compliance with prescribed regimens among members of populations is such that no one can hope to engage all of a randomly chosen sample of a population in a prospective study. Since people who go along with such studies are thought to have characteristics different from those who do not, no prospective study can be said to truly represent a particular population. But when the results of different prospective studies agree, as has often been the case in regard to the major cardiovascular risk factors, errors inherent in population sampling are less of a problem. Epidemiological studies, despite their limitations, have made it possible to predict, with a fairly high degree of accuracy, which groups of people are most likely to develop cardiovascular diseases. The susceptible groups can be identified on the basis of the risk factors that their members possess. A key question that then arises is, Can the susceptible individuals decrease their risk? Here the epidemiological evidence is equivocal, but some evidence suggests that attempts to modify risk factors may pay off.

The risk factor that almost everyone agrees can be modified with beneficial results is high blood pressure (hypertension). It is also one of the best predictors of cardiovascular disease, according to analyses of numerous prospective studies. For example, for participants in a prospective study of people in Framingham, Massachusetts, it was a better predictor than either cigarette smoking or serum cholesterol.

Hypertension is generally defined as blood pressure greater than 160/95 millimeters of mercury. According to this definition, the hypertensive men and women aged 45 to 74 who took part in this study had about three times as much coronary heart disease and over seven times the incidence of brain infarctions as did participants with normal blood pressures. Framingham participants with borderline hypertension, defined as blood pressures greater than 140/90 millimeters of mercury also experienced substantially increased incidences of cardiovascular diseases when compared to those with normal blood pressures. The incidences of these diseases among participants with mild hypertension were intermediate between those of participants with definte hypertension and those with normal blood pressures. The Framingham results are supported by results from other prospective studies, all of which provide evidence that the risk of cardiovascular diseases increases with increasing blood pressure, even for blood pressures within the normal range.

Since 1950, drugs that significantly reduce high blood pressure have been available. Evidence that those who take these drugs may also decrease their risk of developing cardiovascular diseases comes from the Veterans Administration Cooperative Study on Hypertensive Agents, coordinated by Martin Edwards Freis. Veterans (mainly middle-aged men) with definite hypertension who were treated had a significantly reduced incidence of stroke, heart failure, and renal failure when compared to a similar group of veterans who did not take the drugs. Although the population in this study is not representative of the subpopulation in the United States that has high blood pressure (for example, women, who are more prone than men to develop hypertension, are not represented), results lead most researchers to conclude that antihypertensive drugs are highly effective in reducing risks of cardiovascular diseases.

Cigarette smoking has repeatedly been shown to increase substantially the risk of cardiovascular disease, and there is some evidence that those who stop smoking may decrease their risk. The Framingham Study indicates, for example, that men who smoked at the beginning of the study and subsequently stopped had only half as many heart attacks after 18 years as those who continued to smoke.

Two studies far larger than the Framingham Study led to similar conclusions about the effects of giving up cigarettes. About 300,000 U.S. veterans were studied for 8.5 years by Eugene Rogot and his associates at NHLBI. They found that the mortality rates of cigarette smokers were 1.6 times those of nonsmokers. The risk was related to the number of cigarettes smoked. For example, persons who smoke more than 40 cigarettes per day and are between the ages of 30 and 34 have increased their risk almost threefold. The risk for those who stopped smoking decreased with the time since they last smoked.

A second large-scale study was undertaken by the ACS under the direction of E. Cuyler Hammond. These investigators monitored over 1 million people for 6 years by questionnaire. The results indicated that the mortality rate from coronary disease for those who had smoked more than 20 cigarettes a day and who had not smoked for at least 20 years was almost the same as that of those who had never smoked. There are problems in the design of these studies, but since they all lead to similar conclusions, most investigators believe that the results apply to the population at large.

Changes in serum cholesterol concentrations and their effects on the risk of developing cardiovascular diseases are just as difficult to study as changes in blood pressure or smoking habits. One unresolved question is, Can serum cholesterol concentrations be safely, easily, and effectively decreased by drugs? Some drugs are available, but it is not clear whether it is safe to take them for long periods of time or whether they are effective. The NHLBI clinical trial designed to see whether these drugs can effectively lower serum cholesterol concentrations and decrease incidences of heart disease in a select group of men is now under way, but the results will not be available for years.

Diet alone has often been suggested as a means of reducing serum cholesterol concentrations and, possibly, the risk of cardiovascular disease, but epidemiological studies are not sufficient to support the hypothesis that changes in diet decrease the risk. In most studies in which investigators have tried to determine whether a low-fat, low-cholesterol diet does decrease blood cholesterol concentrations and the risk of coronary heart disease, only modest — approximately 10 percent — reductions in blood cholesterol have been observed; the data were not adequate to show whether this reduction affected coronary mortality. In fact, there is no consensus among researchers as to whether the evidence that diet affects serum cholesterol concentrations and subsequent risks of cardiovascular disease is strong enough so that most people in the United States should be persuaded to modify what they eat. One problem with advocating diets low in saturated fats and cholesterol is that many people will substitute carbohydrates for fats. But high carbohydrate diets have adverse effects on some people.

Epidemiological evidence that diet affects serum cholesterol concentrations and risk of heart disease is usually impossible to obtain from studies of any one population. The people of a given country often vary so little in their dietary habits that it cannot be demonstrated that those who develop heart disease eat different foods from those who do not develop heart disease. However, people of different countries may vary substantially in their eating habits and do experience different rates of heart disease. This was illustrated by several studies, including the International Cooperative Study on the Epidemiology of Cardiovascular Disease, a prospective study of 18 population samples in seven countries—Finland, Greece, Italy, Japan, the Netherlands, the United States, and Yugoslavia.

In that study, which extended over a 10-year period, investigators compared the incidence of heart disease among 12,000 men who were between 40 and 59 years of age at the beginning of the study. Mean rates of heart disease varied fourfold with the highest rates in the United States and Finland and the lowest in Japan. The rates were significantly correlated with the serum cholesterol concentrations and also with the saturated fat intake of the populations. Other components of the diets, which included total calories, total fat, monounsaturated fat, polyunsaturated fat, and total protein, were not significantly correlated with incidences of heart disease.

Since different populations have different genetic backgrounds and different life-styles, the independent effects of diet and cholesterol are hard to assess. This is a problem that applies to all studies that examine relationships between diet, cholesterol, and heart disease. Those investigators who advocate changes in diet generally do not say that epidemiological evidence proves that diet will be effective. Instead, they draw on biochemical studies of heart disease in animals and in humans to support that contention.

Several investigators have shown that when primates and other laboratory animals are fed diets high in saturated fats and cholesterol they develop plaques that resemble atherosclerotic plaques in humans. Although these observations do not prove that the same thing happens in humans, Stamler cautions against supposing that humans are different from all other animals, including primates. Further, it may be significant that certain human genetic disorders which produce very high concentrations of serum cholesterol also produce coronary heart disease at an early age. These disorders cannot yet be successfully treated by diet therapy, but they do demonstrate that a very high concentration of serum cholesterol is associated with heart disease. While admitting that no one piece of evidence by itself proves anything, many investigators believe that all the evidence, considered as a whole, shows a plausible, if not certain, link between diet, serum cholesterol, and heart disease.

Obtaining convincing epidemiological evidence that changes in blood pressure, smoking habits, or serum cholesterol concentrations can change the risk of developing cardiovascular diseases is difficult enough, but investigating the effects of changes in other human behavior patterns is even more difficult. For example, most researchers believe that people who exercise have decreased their risk of developing cardiovascular disease, but studies have not as yet substantiated that belief.

In sum, epidemiology has suggested possible causes of cardiovascular diseases, but it has not provided proof that the various conditions identified as correlates actually cause these diseases. These suggested causes are, however, guides to further investigations by the biochemists and clinicians who are attempting to paint a general picture of the causes and pathogenesis of cardiovascular diseases. Through such studies, it is hoped that prevention, amelioration, or even cures may be found.

3

CLINICAL TRIALS
Methodological and Ethical Questions

The second half of this century is the age of the clinical trial. Or so says Jeremiah Stamler of Northwestern University Medical School. Clinical trials are not only coming into increasing use but are becoming increasingly sophisticated and increasingly costly, and many now involve enormous numbers of participants.

These trends are especially notable in clinical trials involving heart disease. The National Heart, Lung, and Blood Institute (NHLBI) is currently devoting a large portion of its research budget to these trials. Some trials are testing whether proposed means to prevent heart disease, such as lowering blood pressure and serum cholesterol concentrations or stopping cigarette smoking, are actually effective. Other trials are testing whether treatments of heart disease currently in use do indeed decrease mortality rates. Some of these treatments are coronary bypass surgery, aspirin, and drugs (such as propranolol) given to patients within the first 18 hours after a heart attack to prevent further damage to the heart. However, those who plan and conduct clinical trials of treatments such as these must be concerned with more than the probable efficacy of the particular treatment. They must deal not only with the methodological problems inherent in any very large, very costly trial but also with the ethical complications which arise whenever trials must involve human participants.

A decision to start a large-scale clinical trial is a decision to commit a great deal of money and effort over a long period of time — often as long as a decade — in the hope of deciding whether a treatment or preventive measure is worthwhile. For various reasons, not all clinical trials are successful, and possible failures of large trials are becoming a bone of contention among medical scientists.

What irks some critics of clinical trials is that certain trials seem to have been initiated for political reasons. For example, the NHLBI has been pressured to come out in favor of cholesterol-lowering diets to prevent heart disease. However, according to Basil Rifkind of the Lipid Research Clinic of the NHLBI, there is no direct evidence in humans that these diets are worthwhile. The NHLBI therefore has begun a clinical trial that bears on the diet-heart disease question. For financial and logistical reasons, this trial necessarily involved methodological compromises and has been criticized for this reason.

The trial, which is directed by the Lipid Research Clinic (LRC), is specifically designed to determine whether lowering blood cholesterol concentrations can prevent heart disease. Rifkind, who is head of the LRC, says that if the LRC trial demonstrates that cholesterol lowering prevents heart disease, he and Robert Levy, head of the NHLBI would be prepared to advocate a national program to change peoples' diets and thereby decrease their blood cholesterol concentrations. However, there is disagreement about whether the current trial can possibly produce the data that would be needed to back such a position.

One major difficulty in obtaining adequate data from clinical trials concerns the ethical responsibilities of the investigators to the participants. Looking back on their experiences with the NHLBI clinical trials and other trials, medical researchers are asking whether certain trials should be conducted at all and, if so, when. Further problems arise once trials are under way, not the least of which is to decide when to end a trial. Often one group of trial participants seems to be harmed by a treatment being tested. If this occurs, some researchers argue, the trial should be ended for ethical reasons, even before statistically significant results are obtained. Others say that certain trials have been ended too soon and thus their results will always be under question. No hard and fast answers to such problems arising from clinical trials are likely to be forthcoming, but some changing trends in researchers' attitudes toward trials are apparent. As a byproduct, this questioning is bringing to the fore avid discussions of medical ethics.

According to Robert Levine of Yale University School of Medicine and Karen Labacqz of the Pacific School of Religion in Berkeley, California, a conference on clinical trial methodology held at the

National Institutes of Health on 3 and 4 October 1977 was actually "all about ethics." They point out that most people assume that the major ethical issue relating to clinical trials involves how to obtain informed consent. However, a question such as, When should a clinical trial be stopped?, "is an ethical question that cannot be resolved by looking only to scientific considerations," they said. Researchers must consider the possibility of harming trial participants as well as that of harming patients waiting for the development of new treatments. Similar ethical issues underlie all aspects of the design and execution of trials involving humans.

Despite the controversy surrounding many trials, the scientific merits of randomized, controlled clinical trials are generally acknowledged. In these trials participants are assigned at random to treatment and control groups. One group is given a new or experimental treatment; the control groups gets conventional treatment or a placebo. The randomization is designed to average out possibly pertinent differences among the trial participants, such as age, sex, and general state of health. (The variables that are pertinent are usually not known.) The treatment and control groups, then, should be medically equivalent.

Unfortunately, among the most difficult trials to design, and the most controversial, are those testing various ways to prevent chronic diseases such as heart disease. For example, designers of trials testing treatments of heart disease must contend with the fact that an average of only one out of every 100 middle-aged men suffers a heart attack each year. To see whether a particular preventive measure decreases rates of heart attacks in the general population of middle-aged men would require more resources than the government or any private organization has available. Trials for new treatments are less expensive than prevention trials and require fewer participants. For example, in a trial designed to test ways of treating heart attack patients, the participants would have already developed heart disease and so would be more likely to die of heart attacks in the near future than members of the general population.

Many researchers believe that trials testing preventive measures must still be conducted, even if the trial designs must be compromised in order to make them feasible. For example, the ideal way to run a trial on cholesterol and heart disease would be to randomly assign trial participants to two groups. Members of one group would follow their normal diets and members of the other group would follow a cholesterol-lowering diet. This sort of trial cannot be conducted, however, for even if compliance with the diets could be ensured, the trial would involve far too many people for far too long a time before any effects could be seen. In fact, in 1969 a National Institutes of Health study group concluded that such a trial would require 50,000 to 100,000 people, 30 years of follow-up, and could cost as much as $1 billion.

As an expedient, the LRC designed a trial whose participants are men with cholesterol concentrations within the top 5 percent of the normal distribution in this country. Because the designers of this trial found that it would take too many participants and too much time if diet alone were used to lower cholesterol, they decided to use the drug cholestyramine to lower the participants' cholesterol concentrations more significantly. Diet, Rifkind points out, can only reduce cholesterol concentrations by 5 to 10 percent. Thus the treatment group is given cholestyramine and a cholesterol-lowering diet. The control group is given the same diet but is given a placebo instead of the drug. The trial involves 3600 men, will continue for 7 years, and is expected to cost more than $100 million.

Proponents of the LRC trial argue that the trial is worthwhile because prevention, not treatment, is the key to lowering the toll taken by heart disease. Thomas Chalmers of Mt. Sinai Medical Center says that the cost of a prevention trial must be compared to the cost of medical care rather than to the cost of doing other kinds of research. Each day a patient spends in a coronary care unit, he says, costs about $1000. And there are about 1 million heart attacks each year in the United States. (Although many of these heart attack victims die before they ever reach the hospital, Chalmers points out that those who die represent a significant economic loss to the country.)

Critics of the prevention trials contend that the trials would undoubtedly be worthwhile if they indeed showed that particular preventive measures were useful and if people then employed those measures. But a trial such as the LRC trial, they say, can at best have only a marginal effect in preventing heart disease. After years of public education campaigns by the American Heart Association and others, many people in the United States are already convinced that cholesterol-lowering diets will prevent heart disease. (Not all of these people, however, are sufficiently motivated to follow such diets.) Those who are still skeptical of the diet-heart disease hypothesis may be unlikely to change their minds on the basis of the LRC study. Thus even a positive result from the LRC trial could be a mere whistling in the wind.

George Mann of Vanderbilt University, a forceful critic of the diet-heart disease hypothesis, reports that he has received letters of support for his criticism from 40 to 50 leaders of the American medical establishment. Mann says he would not be convinced of the diet-heart disease hypothesis by positive results from the LRC trial. He believes that the LRC results could not be extrapolated to the general population because they involve a select group of high-risk men who are not representative of the rest of the U.S. population. Moreover, cholesterol is being lowered with a drug, not by a diet alone, which further confounds the results.

According to Mann, at least one planner of an NHLBI prevention trial admits privately that the trial he is involved with cannot produce meaningful results. But, Mann says, the planners of these prevention trials "get so involved in obtaining financial support that they'll do and say just about anything to keep their trials going."

Closely related to the problem of deciding whether to start a randomized, controlled clinical trial is the problem of deciding when such a trial should begin. Usually, a randomized controlled trial is suggested on the basis of presumptive evidence that a particular treatment or preventive measure is useful. However, Chalmers estimates that fewer than 20 percent of trials testing new therapies of any kind are well controlled. And this percentage can be far smaller than 20. A few years ago, Chalmers surveyed the clinical-trial abstracts submitted to the annual meeting of the American Gastroenterological Association. He noted that only 4.5 percent of those trials appeared to be well-controlled.

Many physicians prescribe treatments on the basis of results from uncontrolled or poorly controlled studies. They often come to believe in the efficacy of those treatments and feel ethically constrained from allowing their patients to participate in randomized controlled trials. They cannot in good conscience risk denying a patient what they believe to be the best treatment, even if their belief is not scientifically justified.

Clinical investigators are often in a quandary when they must decide when to start a randomized controlled trial. To start when a great deal of presumptive evidence favoring a treatment has been published is to risk fighting physicians who already believe in the treatment. To start too soon is to risk wasting years and a great deal of money testing a treatment that, by the time the trial results are out, has been modified, replaced, or discarded by practicing physicians. Both of these difficulties arose when investigators planned randomized controlled trials of the effects of coronary bypass surgery.

Recently, investigators at the NHLBI initiated a randomized controlled trial to compare the effects of coronary bypass surgery to the effects of drugs on the longevity of patients with certain forms of angina pectoris, which are chest pains arising from atherosclerosis. A large number of poorly controlled studies had already been published, most of which indicated that surgery prolongs the lives of these patients. As a result, many cardiologists and surgeons are already convinced that it would be unethical to deny their patients what they believe are the life-prolonging benefits of surgery. These physicians not only are not participating in the NHLBI study, but some say they will not accept the trials' results unless surgery is vindicated.

The Veterans Administration (VA) decided a decade ago to study the effects of bypass surgery on the mortality of patients with angina pectoris. In 1968, when the VA began its randomized controlled trial, the Vineberg procedure was the operation of choice. In this procedure, clogged coronary arteries are bypassed with internal mammary arteries. Soon after the VA trial began, the Vineberg procedure was replaced by the operation still popular today – a bypass that makes use of a vein from the patient's leg. The VA then had to redesign its trial to study the vein bypass instead. Thus it can be argued that the VA started its trial too soon and that the NHLBI may have started its trial too late.

Once a randomized controlled trial is under way, investigators often see trends in the accumulating data that make them ask whether the trial should be halted. These trends may indicate that a particular treatment may be harmful or that a treatment may be beneficial or that one treatment may be more harmful than another. At this point they are faced with a difficult ethical question. If they end the trial before they obtain statistically significant results, they run the risk of failing to discover the best treatment because they will never know whether the suspected hazardous or helpful treatment is actually as good or bad as it appears to be. If they wait too long to end the trial, the patients involved may suffer needlessly.

Just how significant these decisions can be is shown by one trial conducted by the NHLBI which was, at least partially, prematurely terminated. The trial was the Coronary Drug Project (CDP)—a randomized study designed to see whether drugs that lower peoples' serum cholesterol concentrations can increase the life-spans of heart attack patients. The study tested five different drugs and a placebo.

Three of the drugs soon seemed to be causing serious side effects and did not seem to be prolonging the participants' lives. For example, individuals in the group treated with estrogen—one of the drugs tested—had increased incidences of pulmonary embolisms. The trial designers then decided to terminate tests with the three treatment groups that seemingly were being harmed, even though there was not yet evidence of whether these drugs did or did not prevent heart attacks. "It was a difficult decision," says Lawrence Friedman of the NHLBI, but the trial overseers believed that any possible beneficial effects of these drugs could not outweigh the known harmful ones.

The two remaining drugs tested in the CDP trial—clofibrate and niacin—did not seem to be seriously harming the trial participants. They produced modest reductions (an average of less than 10 percent) in the participants' serum cholesterol concentrations but did have some unpleasant or moderately hazardous side effects, such as disturbances of heart rhythms. Finally, after the trial participants had taken these drugs or a placebo for a total of 5 to 8 years, the CDP was ended. The conclusion was that neither niacin nor clofibrate significantly increased the survivals of the participants when compared to a placebo.

The decision to partially terminate the CDP trial ahead of schedule was less controversial than some other decisions to end clinical trials.

According to Paul Meier of the University of Chicago, the current trend is to terminate a trial when there is some evidence that a treatment is harmful, even when that evidence is not statistically significant. In the past, the tendency was to continue until significant results were obtained.

Such troublesome decisions are by no means limited to clinical trials on heart diseases, but are endemic to all such studies involving humans. In discussing this problem, Meier mentions several other examples of studies that were ended prematurely for ethical reasons, to the detriment of the studies' conclusions. One example involves

clinical trials comparing the effects of simple and radical mastectomies on the survival of breast cancer patients. Meier contrasts two
studies, both of which were terminated prematurely, that came to
opposite conclusions. The first of these studies was conducted in
Cambridge, England, and was terminated when an early trend in
the results seemed to favor simple mastectomies. The decision to end
the study was made because the trial's designers felt that it was
unlikely that radical mastectomies would improve the patients'
survivals. Meier stated that, "Nothing was yet significant, and a
decision was reached, not on the grounds of evidence about a true
difference, but on grounds of evidence about a future significance
level."

A similar study of mastectomies was conducted in London, but
this trial was terminated prematurely in favor of radical mastectomies. As Meier said, "Once again, results at the bare margin of
statistical significance were deemed to require cutting off the study
on ethical grounds."

Still another trial that was ended prematurely has actually led
to a lawsuit. This trial, conducted by the University Group Diabetes
Project (UGDP), was designed to determine whether oral hypergly-
cemic drugs can delay retinal damage, liability to infection, and
other complications of adult-onset diabetes. The study was ended
when it appeared that some of the drugs might cause excessive
mortality from heart disease. The UGDP investigators concluded
that the benefits of these drugs, if any, could not outweigh this risk.
Still, said Meier, it was far from certain that the drugs were harmful
and "a great deal in convincingness was lost by not continuing until
the evidence became clearer." Now a group of physicians and drug
companies has brought suit against the UDGP, claiming that patients are being denied possibly beneficial drugs.

Meier discussed a final example of a premature trial termination
to illustrate how investigators often make unconscious value judg-
ments when they end trials. More than 20 years ago, a randomized
controlled study was conducted to determine the effects of the
administration of oxygen to premature infants. Some evidence from
uncontrolled studies had indicated that oxygen might cause a form of
blindness (retrolental fibroplasia) in these infants. Yet the babies
were often gasping for air, and it was believed that oxygen might
save their lives.

When the randomized controlled trial was conducted, investigators found that the infants given oxygen were indeed more likely to become blind. The study was terminated before it could be determined whether the oxygen saved lives as well. Meier pointed out, however, that the decision to terminate the trial was based on a possibly inadvertent judgment about the value of a dead as opposed to a blind baby. "The data [in favor of termination] are conclusive only if you think a dead baby is $2^1/2$ times worse than a blind one," he said.

Each stage of the progress of a randomized controlled clinical trial, from the decision to begin to the decision to end, meets with resistance caused by a combination of social, political, and ethical forces. And finally, the results must face the test of justification: Were they worth the time and money? Clinical investigators hope that their experiences in this age of clinical trials will increase both their awareness of the pitfalls associated with such trials and their knowledge of new ways to avoid the pitfalls. If so, the theoretical advantages of randomized, controlled clinical trials will more likely be reflected in practice.

II

Life-Styles and Heart Disease

4

LIFE-STYLES AND
HEART DISEASE
A Disease of Modern Living

Nearly 1 million people in the United States have heart attacks each year — a number so huge that heart disease must be considered ubiquitous in our society. Most other technologically advanced societies also have high incidences of heart disease, but more primitive societies do not. The !Kung, for example, who have lived as hunter-gatherers in the Kalahari Desert for at least 11,000 years, have very little heart disease. They are also one of only about a dozen groups of people in the world whose blood pressure does not increase as they grow older. Jeremiah Stamler of Northwestern University describes heart disease as "the epidemic disease of a mature, advanced industrial society, as TB was the epidemic disease of this society in its childhood and infancy."

What is it about modern living that predisposes people to develop heart disease? Epidemiologists have noted that, as per capita income increases, diets change. People eat more animal fats and sugar and less grain, for example. Cigarette smoking also increases. At the same time, people become more sedentary, their cardiopulmonary fitness decreases, and they become fatter. Some researchers also believe that stress increases. As Stamler puts it, "the stress, tensions, and conflicts of modern life in highly urbanized society, and the pace, turmoil, mobility, and change and their effects on personality and behavior act as insult added to injury for sizable segments of the populations of advanced countries."

Cross-cultural comparisons have thus provided clues that behavior patterns might be implicated in the current epidemic of heart disease in industrial societies. But following up these clues to discover aspects of modern life-styles that actually cause heart disease is another matter. Many medical scientists firmly believe that cholesterol-lowering diets protect against heart disease. Increased exercise and relaxation are also thought to be protective. Unfortunately, proof of these beliefs is yet to be found.

The question of whether cholesterol-lowering diets protect against heart disease has long been hotly debated. One critic of the diet-heart disease concept, George Mann of Vanderbilt University, describes the past 25 years of research on the subject as "the lost generation of misguided and fruitless preoccupation with the diet-heart hypothesis." He claims that investigators were pressured to accept the hypothesis in order to obtain research funds: "To be a dissenter was to be unfunded because the peer-review system rewards conformity and excludes criticism."

Mann points out several reasons for believing that the diet-heart disease hypothesis is wrong. He notes, for example, that there was no correlation between dietary habits and high concentrations of blood cholesterol among 1000 persons in the Framingham Study or among 2000 persons in another study, the Tecumseh Study. Moreover, he says, people in the United States have doubled their intake of unsaturated fats since 1900 but have not increased their intake of saturated fats or cholesterol. During this time, heart disease rates increased dramatically. Clinical trials, he reports, have also failed to demonstrate the diet-heart disease hypothesis.

Proponents of cholesterol-lowering diets argue that epidemiological evidence seems to be in their favor. Populations of countries whose national diets are high in saturated fats tend to have higher blood cholesterol concentrations and proportionately more heart disease than populations of countries whose diets are low in saturated fats. In addition, studies with animals, including primates, indicate that diets high in saturated fats and cholesterol can cause atherosclerosis.

The NHLBI has allegedly been under political pressure to come out in favor of a national policy favoring cholesterol-lowering diets and has initiated a clinical trial that, it hopes, may provide evidence that cholesterol reduction can prevent heart disease in humans. Since this trial has also been criticized on methodological grounds, those such as Mann who have publicly come out against the diet-heart disease hypothesis are unlikely to change their positions because of its results.

At least as difficult to prove or disprove as the diet-heart disease hypothesis are the hypotheses that increased exercise or decreased stress can protect against heart disease. One problem with testing these hypotheses is the difficulty of assessing behavior patterns. Do you ask people how much exercise they get or how tense they feel? If so, the answers may vary from day to day. A man who just started a jogging program, for example, may report that he exercises regularly. A month later, he may have abandoned the program. A woman who recently changed jobs may report that she is under a great deal of stress. But this stress may soon diminish.

Investigators have attempted to conduct "intervention" studies of life-styles and heart disease. In these studies, a group of people agree to participate in regular exercise or behavior modification sessions. Their incidences of heart disease are then compared to those of control groups. These intervention studies, however, have failed to yield convincing results. J. N. Morris of the London School of Hygiene analyzes their failure by saying, "It's not a question of problems of knowledge, politics, or even finance. The sheer technical difficulties of these intervention studies are such that, although we know in theory how to do them, they do not work out in practice."

Some researchers conclude that it may never be known to what extent, if any, proposed changes in life-styles may prevent heart disease. They also recognize that, even if the proposed changes were proved beneficial, many people would be unwilling or unable to change their behavior accordingly. Nonetheless, many of these medical researchers as well as members of the general public are adhering to exercise programs and following cholesterol-lowering diets, and some are even using biofeedback techniques to learn to relax. Many of those who realize that there is no proof that these changes in life-style will prevent heart disease would undoubtedly agree with Irvine Page, a cardiologist at the Cleveland Clinic. Page explains his adherence to a cholesterol-lowering diet by saying he has no intention of being the smartest man in the graveyard.

5

STRESS AND PERSONALITY
Their Role in Cardiovascular Disease

Despite decades of effort, medical scientists have failed to pinpoint the causes of coronary heart disease (CHD) and hypertension. The problem is that several different factors are now thought to contribute to the development of the diseases, but the interactions between these contributing factors are not as yet understood. Moreover, there may be other factors as yet unidentified. For example, epidemiologists have associated a number of risk factors, such as smoking and high concentrations of blood cholesterol, with an increased likelihood of developing CHD. However, not everyone in whom the risk factors are present suffers a heart attack, and many people who do have heart attacks are not members of the high-risk groups. The situation regarding the causes of hypertension is even more confused.

Because the risk factors identified thus far have not provided a full explanation for the massive incidence of cardiovascular diseases in this and many other highly developed countries, investigators are still looking for conditions, including psychological factors, that may predispose individuals to the diseases. Stress is one such factor which has long been suspect. It is generally accepted as a risk factor by both the press and the public, although not necessarily by the medical profession. Articles appearing in such popular magazines as *Business Week* and *Psychology Today* advocate changes in life-style to decrease stress on the premise that this will prevent heart attacks or lower blood pressure.

But just how firm is the evidence providing the basis for these recommendations? There are studies indicating that people with a high degree of stress in their lives are at higher risk of developing a wide spectrum of diseases, including those of the heart and circulatory system. However, some experts in epidemiology recently concluded that studies have thus far failed to establish a clear link between stress and the development of hypertension. And as yet, no one has ever shown that avoidance of stress can actually decrease the incidence of either chronic high blood pressure or CHD. Thus, many medical scientists think that recommendations of drastic changes in life-style are still premature.

Stress can be defined in two ways. By one definition, stress is an external event or environment that elicits a particular set of physiological responses—the "fight, flight, or fright" reaction—in an individual. By the other definition, it is the psychological and physiological changes produced in the person responding. How people respond to various events may be at least partially determined by their personalities and characteristic behavior patterns. Thus, some investigators have searched for external events that might be linked with a higher incidence of CHD or hypertension, while others have looked at personal characteristics that might predispose only certain individuals to develop such diseases. A third approach has been to try to identify the physiological mechanisms by which stress may produce pathological responses.

Heart attacks and CHD have been linked to a specific behavior pattern—the type A, or coronary-prone personality—by Meyer Friedman and Ray Rosenman of Mount Zion Hospital and Medical Center in San Francisco. They have characterized the type A individual as marked by excessive time-urgency, impatience, competitiveness, aggression, and hostility. As a result, the type A person is often in a state of internal stress that may be largely self-imposed and not necessary for coping with the environment. (Although Friedman and Rosenman have studied mainly men, women can also have type A personalities.) Persons lacking the type A characteristics are said to be type B and, according to Friedman and Rosenman, are at a lower risk of having heart attacks. There is growing—but not universal—acceptance by the medical community of the type A behavior pattern as a risk factor for CHD.

In their first study, carried out almost 20 years ago, Friedman and Rosenman identified 83 type A men and 83 type B men in the community. They then determined that 28 percent of the type A men, but only 4 percent of the type B men, had suffered heart attacks. In the intervening years, additional epidemiological studies performed by other investigators appeared to confirm the existence of a possible link between personality and heart attacks. However, many of these studies have been retrospective in nature and have been criticized for that reason.

In a retrospective study, heart or other patients are questioned about events that occurred in their lives before they became ill. Their responses are compared with those of healthy persons or patients with illnesses unrelated to the heart. All retrospective studies seeking to establish a link betwen an illness and stress are beset by similar problems in interpretation. If patients, who may have come close to death or who have to cope with a chronic condition for the rest of their lives, do report a higher level of stress than controls, it may only be because sick people are more conscious of stress and are more likely to regard a particular event as stressful than would healthy persons.

However, prospective studies have also shown an association between type A behavior and CHD. One of the largest of these was the Western Collaborative Group Study. It included 3400 men between the ages of 39 and 59 who were apparently free of heart problems when they entered the study in 1960 and 1961. After 8.5 years of follow-up, Friedman, Rosenman, and C. David Jenkins of Boston University Medical School reported that the risk of developing CHD was about twice as great for type A men as for type B men. They observed the increased risk even after they corrected for the contributions of some 12 other CHD risk factors.

In another prospective study, Richard Shekelle and James Schoenberger of Rush Presbyterian-St. Luke's Medical Center and Jeremiah Stamler of Northwestern University Medical School found that the predictive value for CHD of the type A personality rating was slightly better than that of serum cholesterol concentrations but not quite as good as that of diastolic blood pressures. Increased blood cholesterol concentrations and blood pressures are both accepted physical risk factors for the disease.

Furthermore, there is objective evidence that the coronary arteries of type A persons tend to be more severely blocked by atherosclerotic plaques than those of type B persons. Some of the evidence comes from autopsies of individuals who have died. In addition, in two studies, one at Boston University School of Medicine and the other at Duke University Medical Center, there was a strong relation between type A behavior patterns and the severity of atherosclerosis of the coronary arteries of patients undergoing angiography for suspected coronary artery disease.

The work of Friedman and Rosenman has been criticized because they rely on personal interviews to characterize behavior patterns. Until recently, anyone who wanted to learn the interview method had to be taught by Friedman or Rosenman or one of their colleagues. Moreover, interviews tend to be subjective, and apparently not everyone was able to master the technique. Recently, however, Friedman and Rosenman have developed a checklist of some 40 physical signs indicative of type A behavior. The presence or absence of these signs is easily recognized by the interviewer, and the identification of type A individuals has thus become more objective.

In addition, other investigators are trying to develop questionnaires that may be easier to administer than an interview. One of the most widely used was devised by Jenkins. The Jenkins Activity Survey is self-administered and scored by a computer. Comparisons of the results of the questionnaires and interviews with the same respondents indicate that the ratings of the two techniques agree 80 percent of the time in identifying type B persons but that only 65 percent of the type A identifications agree. Friedman says that the lower agreement for type A identification is not surprising because the manner in which a subject responds during an interview is more indicative of his characteristic behavior pattern than what he says. Type A persons exhibit rapid eye movements, knee-jiggling, jaw-clenching, explosive speech, and other mannerisms not observed in type B persons. A questionnaire cannot detect this nonverbal behavior.

Independent corroboration for the existence of the type A personality comes from the work of David Glass, now at the City University of New York. Glass used a modified version of the Jenkins Activity Survey to identify college students as either type A or type B. The students then took a battery of psychological tests to determine whether the two types exhibited differences in responses consistent with the behavior patterns described by Friedman and Rosenman. And they did. For example, type A individuals did not do as well as type B's on a task in which success required that they make a delayed response. Because type A persons are impatient, they could not wait the required interval and responded prematurely. This behavior would be expected of persons who feel a strong sense of time urgency. Glass says that these and other findings provide evidence for the validity of the measures used to classify individuals as type A or B.

Determining a statistical correlation between a risk factor and a disease is only part of the problem that must be solved if the etiology of the disease is to be understood. Also needed is a mechanism that explains how the factor contributes to the development of the pathological changes. Although Friedman and Rosenman have found that type A men have higher concentrations of blood cholesterol than type B men, they do not think that the sterol is the main culprit in the development of CHD. Instead they think that the culprit is excess production of the hormones norepinephrine and adrenocorticotropic hormone. Both of these substances are normally secreted in response to stress, but Friedman and Rosenman have evidence that type A men secrete more of them than type B men in a stressful test situation.

These hormones are suspect because they have profound effects on the cardiovascular system. They increase the blood pressure and the rate and force of the heartbeat, and stimulate platelet aggregation. The latter phenomenon has been implicated in the formation of atherosclerotic plaques. Thus, in the view of Friedman and Rosenman, excess production of the hormones might contribute to the development of the plaques and consequent CHD.

One reason why most cardiologists have been unenthusiastic about personality as a risk factor for CHD is that they were—and still are—pessimistic that anything can be done to modify the personality and thus prevent the disease. Now, however, some investigators are beginning to develop behavior modification programs to help type A persons change their ways and, they hope, reduce their chances of having a heart attack. It is still too early to tell whether the behavior changes will be maintained long after therapy is stopped or if the changes can accomplish the goal of decreasing the incidence of heart attacks.

Moreover, the task of behavior modification seems formidable. To begin with, there are a lot of type A people. Friedman says that about 80 percent of the government employees they are now testing are type A persons. And, although most of the studies done thus far have focused on men, women—both those who work outside the home and those who do not—can have type A personalities, too. Preliminary evidence from Suzanne Haynes of the NHLBI and Ingrid Waldron of the University of Pennsylvania indicates that type A women have a risk of CHD about twice that of type B women. In addition, type A people do not like to take the time to attend therapy sessions unless they have already had a heart attack. That tends to be a powerful motivator.

Richard Suinn of Colorado State University is one of the investigators who has developed a behavior modification program for type A persons. His first two studies involved small groups of heart attack patients (10 in the first study and 17 in the second). According to Suinn, in comparison with a similar group of patients who did not have the therapy, the patients who underwent the 5-week therapy course reported a marked decrease in the stress and anxiety they experienced. He concedes, however, that the decreased anxiety might have been due to the extra attention received by the experimental groups and not to modification of their behavior. But he points out that the blood cholesterol and triglyceride concentrations of the experimental groups also decreased significantly. These results are in line with reports by Friedman and Rosenman that cholesterol concentrations increase during times of stress and decrease when the stress is relieved.

More recently, Suinn has attempted behavior modification with persons who show no signs of CHD. He observed no decreases in their blood cholesterol or triglyceride concentrations, although he points out that these individuals did not eat low-fat, low-cholesterol diets as both the control and experimental groups did in the earlier studies. He did observe a small, but not statistically significant, decrease in the blood pressures of the individuals undergoing behavior modification. They also showed some decrease in type A behavior as assessed by the Jenkins Activity Survey. Suinn did not follow any of the patients or healthy persons studied after the therapy sessions ended and thus does not know how long—or even if—they were able to maintain their modified behavior.

Friedman says that his own experience with patients who have had at least one heart attack has convinced him that behavior modification can pay off in a reduced rate of heart attack recurrence. But his sample size is small and not sufficient to convince most members of the medical profession. With Carl Thoresen of Stanford

University, Friedman is now recruiting 900 type A patients who have had at least one heart attack for a controlled clinical trial of behavior modification.

Bernard Lown of Harvard Medical School is one of the cardiologists who is not convinced that a type A behavior pattern is a risk factor for CHD, but he does think that stress may predispose an individual to the kind of cardiac arrhythmias — ventricular fibrillation, for example — that can culminate in sudden death. Sudden death may be attributed to a heart attack, but, strictly speaking, a heart attack always produces permanent destruction of a portion of the heart muscle as a result of blockage of the coronary arteries, whereas a person may experience ventricular fibrillation and die suddenly even without apparent damage to the heart muscle. The coronary arteries usually show some sign of blockage, however, in persons who have succumbed to sudden death.

According to Lown, stress, acting through the sympathetic nervous system, may help to trigger ventricular fibrillation. He and his colleagues found that, in dogs, either direct stimulation of the sympathetic nervous system or exposure to stress increases the ease with which ventricular fibrillation can be triggered. Recently, they also demonstrated that procedures that increase the concentration of serotonin in the brain decrease the susceptibility of dogs to ventricular fibrillation. Other investigators have shown that increasing brain serotonin decreases the flow of sympathetic nerve impulses to the heart. Lown says that these findings may make it possible to devise drug therapies for the prevention of sudden death that act by suppressing the flow to the heart of sympathetic nerve impulses that might otherwise trigger ventricular fibrillation.

The relationship of stress to hypertension is also of concern, not only because hypertension is a risk factor for atherosclerosis and CHD but because it is also a disease in its own right. People with chronically elevated blood pressures suffer an increased risk of strokes and heart and kidney failure. While medical scientists can usually control hypertension with drugs or diet, they still do not know what causes some 90 percent of the cases they treat.

The belief that stress may cause hypertension is widespread. The theory is that prolonged or repeated exposures to stress may produce permanent physiological changes in some persons who consequently develop chronic hypertension. The difficulty lies in proving that this supposition is correct. As Adrian Ostfeld of Yale

University Medical School puts it: "As a physician who saw patients weekly in the clinic, I was sure that stress could cause hypertension; but as an epidemiologist following patients at 6-month intervals I lost that assurance."

Not in question is the unfavorable effect stress may have on the course of hypertension once it begins. Stress, which can cause transient increases in blood pressure even in normal individuals, may drive elevated pressures even higher, thus accelerating blood vessel damage or even precipitating a stroke in someone with uncontrolled high blood pressure.

Evidence that stress may play a role in the development of hypertension comes from studies of both animals and humans. Investigators in several laboratories have shown that persistent elevations of blood pressure occur in experimental animals exposed to some – but not all – kinds of stress. For example, J. Alan Herd and his associates at Harvard Medical School produced prolonged increases in the blood pressures of squirrel monkeys by submitting them to many daily sessions of an operant conditioning procedure. During the conditioning sessions, the monkeys were sometimes subjected to an electric shock when a light was on. The monkeys could turn off the light and avoid the shock by pressing a lever the required number of times. As the conditioning progressed, they would press the lever whenever the light was on, even though shocks were not always administered.

During the first training sessions, the monkeys' blood pressures were elevated only while the light was on. But after many days of training, Herd found that their pressures remained high before, during, and after each session even if no shocks at all were administered.

Even more striking were the results of stress experiments conducted by James Henry and his colleagues at the School of Medicine of the University of California at Los Angeles. These investigators observed sustained blood pressure increases in mice kept in crowded conditions where they had to compete for living space – a situation similar to urban environments that some studies have linked with an increased risk of hypertension in humans.

Most of the attempts to pin down the role of psychosocial factors in the development of human hypertension have depended on retrospective epidemiological studies subject to all the criticisms usually leveled at retrospective investigations of any kind. Moreover, some epidemiologists are troubled by the inconsistencies they see in the data. One of them, S. Leonard Syme of the University of California at Berkeley, says that "every one of the hypotheses presented by psychosocial epidemiologists regarding the etiology of essential hypertension is contradicted by as much evidence as exists in its support."

As examples, Syme cites some studies that have reported higher blood pressures in urban populations than in rural ones, whereas other studies have found the opposite. (Urban areas are supposed to be more stressful places to live than rural environments.) Even relationships generally thought to be well established may not be as clearcut as they once appeared. The incidence of hypertension is supposed to be higher in women than in men, when the data from all age groups are combined, and higher in blacks than in whites (Figure

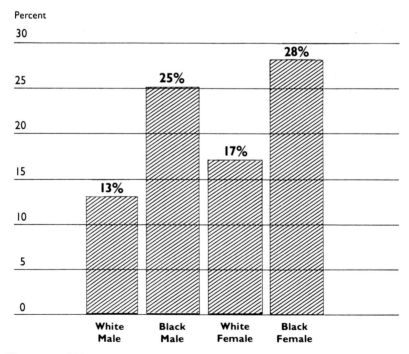

Figure 7. Hypertension prevalence by race and sex in U.S. adults age 20 and over in 1975. [© Reprinted with the permission of the American Heart Association]

7). But most investigations have actually shown that the blood pressures of younger women are usually lower than those of younger men; sometime around the age of 45, the situation reverses.

Moreover, Syme has evidence that socioeconomic class may account for much of the apparent higher incidence of hypertension among blacks than whites. Analysis of data from some 22,000 persons, most of whom are members of the Kaiser Foundation Health Plan in the San Francisco area, indicates that the blood pressures of the members of both races increase as their socioeconomic class decreases. Thus, whatever the cause, members of lower socioeconomic classes appear to be at increased risk of developing chronic high blood pressure. Since a higher proportion of blacks in the United States belongs to the lower socioeconomic classes, the incidence of the condition is higher among blacks than among whites. However, there are studies that have not found a higher incidence of high blood pressure in the lower socioeconomic classes, and these may serve as a further indicator of the confusion surrounding the etiology of hypertension.

The epidemiologists who are dismayed by the failure of their discipline to establish a clear link between stress and hypertension point to a number of possible explanations. One of the most important, according to Richard S. Lazarus of the University of California at Berkeley, is the lack of recognition that stress is an interaction of a particular person with a particular environment. Not every individual will appraise and react to a situation in the same way. One will see it as a challenge to conquer, another as a threat from which to flee, and a third may simply withdraw. If the psychological responses differ, then the physiological reactions might also differ. Lazarus says that few studies have included consideration of these individual variations.

In addition, he maintains that a person's responses vary from time to time, even from moment to moment, and that this variability is not studied in most epidemiological research. Large numbers of people are included in the studies and their physical and psychological states are assessed only infrequently, and sometimes just once. Lazarus thinks that it is possible to gain significant information by studying fewer people more intensively than is usually done and is taking that tack in his own research. By repeatedly measuring the psychological and physiological responses of individuals in varying life situations, he hopes to spot the characteristics of persons at greater risk and to clarify the role of stress—if there is one—in producing chronically elevated blood pressures.

Even if they cannot agree on the causes of hypertension, investigators do agree that there are large differences in individual susceptibilities to the condition. A great deal of effort is currently aimed at identifying those persons who are at higher risk. Particular attention has been focused on individuals with borderline or labile hypertension because there is evidence that these persons may eventually develop a more severe form of the disease. The blood pressures of borderline hypertensives are slightly above normal but lower than those for which drug therapies are ordinarily prescribed. In addition, they may increase dramatically in response to stimuli that have little effect on the blood pressures of normal persons or in situations that should have little effect, such as a visit to the doctor's office.

A view currently gaining acceptance is that mild or borderline hypertension in at least some patients is the result of increased release of norepinephrine by the sympathetic nervous system. Investigators, such as Stevo Julius and his colleagues at the University of Michigan Medical Center, have demonstrated that norepinephrine concentrations are increased in the blood of individuals with mild hypertension and high plasma renin activity. (Renin is an enzyme that produces angiotensin, a very potent increaser of blood pressure.) In these patients, norepinephrine apparently increases blood pressure by stimulating cardiac output and increasing peripheral resistance to blood flow. Although renin itself might increase blood pressure, Julius says that he and his colleagues have found evidence indicating that the production of the enzyme is secondary to norepinephrine production and is not the cause of the elevated blood pressures.

According to Julius, psychological testing of individuals with mild hypertension and high plasma renin activity indicates that they show increased levels of anxiety and suppressed hostility compared to normal controls and other hypertension patients. Anger is known to increase blood pressures, at least transiently, by activating the sympathetic nervous system. Julius hypothesizes that the pathogenesis of the blood pressure elevation in these patients may involve suppression of hostility as a persistent behavior pattern, leading to chronic activation of the sympathetic nervous system. But he concedes that the increased sympathetic nervous activity might be the cause rather than the effect of suppressed hostility. Norepinephrine is a neurotransmitter in the brain, too, and its overproduction might affect mood.

Several investigators in addition to Julius have suggested that there is a "hypertensive personality" characterized by a high degree of suppressed anger and "tendermindedness" (meaning an increased tendency to develop hurt feelings). However, not everyone has observed these traits in hypertensive patients, and the issue is still in doubt. The possibility that the hypertensive personality may actually be associated only with some subgroups of patients may help to account for the inconsistent findings.

Paul Obrist of the University of North Carolina Medical School is another investigator who is focusing on the interaction between stress and the sympathetic nervous system in the development of hypertension. Although most earlier studies have emphasized the role of sympathetic effects that increase peripheral resistance by causing constriction of the blood vessels, Obrist thinks that sympathetic stimulation of the heart, which increases cardiac output, may initially be more important in elevating blood pressures.

Obrist and Kathleen Light, also of the University of North Carolina Medical School, have found, for example, that a stressful situation in which the test subjects have only partial control over the outcome of the experimental events raises the systolic blood pressures of some — but not all — of the subjects. (The systolic pressure is the pressure in the arteries when the heart is contracting.) The investigators think that the most likely explanation for the subjects' elevated systolic pressures is increased cardiac output caused by stress acting on the heart through the sympathetic nervous system. Drugs that block the action of sympathetic neurons on the heart minimize or prevent the increased pressures in the human subjects.

In experiments with dogs, Obrist and Light directly measured cardiac output and tissue oxygen consumption in addition to blood pressure. When the dogs were exposed to a test situation similar to the one producing the response in humans, the cardiac output and systolic blood pressures of the animals increased. These changes were also minimized by the drugs that prevent sympathetic nerve impulses from stimulating the heart. Measurements of tissue oxygen consumption indicated that the extra blood pumped by the heart is in excess of that actually required by the tissues during the test.

Other investigators have suggested that perfusion of the tissues with more blood than they need may be a factor in the development of hypertension. To prevent tissue damage as a result of excessive oxygen concentrations, the vessels to the tissues would constrict to reduce the blood flow. With repeated stimulation of this kind, the artery walls might thicken and the constriction become permanent, thus producing chronically elevated blood pressures.

In their tests with humans, Obrist and Light observed large variations in the way the subjects responded to the test situation in which they had partial control. Some experienced very large blood pressure increases and others none at all. Obrist postulates that the responders may be more likely to develop chronic hypertension in the future; additional studies in which responders and nonresponders are followed for years will be needed to confirm this hypothesis. In addition, he noted that responding to one kind of stimulus did not mean that the same individual would respond to another. Understanding the physiological basis for individual differences such as these may help to determine whether stress, acting through the nervous system, plays a role in the etiology of hypertension.

On the other hand, Ostfeld's investigations at Yale lead him to think that no nervous system mechanism may be required to explain the putative role of stress in producing chronic high blood pressure. He points out that the relationship between excess weight and elevated blood pressures is a most consistently demonstrated linkage. Hypertensive patients tend to be heavier than persons with normal blood pressures. Moreover, persons with normal pressures are less likely to develop hypertension than obese individuals. And when hypertensive individuals lose weight, their blood pressures drop. Another dietary factor, excessive intake of salt, is also widely, if not universally, accepted as predisposing some people to develop hypertension.

According to Ostfeld, stress may lead indirectly to hypertension by increasing appetite and thus the intake of food, including salt. He says that the relationships between sociocultural variables and obesity parallel those between the variables and the incidence of hypertension. For example, many studies have shown that moving from a traditional agricultural or hunting society to an urban environment is associated with an increased incidence of hypertension in the population involved. (Not all studies support this contention, however). This change may be stressful, but it is also usually accompanied by decreased physical activity and increased food consumption, both of which contribute to a gain in weight. Moreover, some studies indicate that the incidence of both obesity and hypertension increase as socioeconomic class decreases in highly developed countries. Thus, Ostfeld says that, in view of the inconsistencies in the data attempting to correlate stress and hypertension, obesity and high salt intake may be more plausible explanations for the development of hypertension than are stress-induced neurological changes. Ostfeld's hypothesis is still controversial, however.

Whatever causes hypertension, several investigators, including Herbert Benson of Harvard Medical School and Gary Schwartz of Yale University, have shown that various "relaxation" and biofeedback techniques can produce modest decreases in the blood pressures of hypertensive patients. The decreases produced by these methods may persist and not just be limited to the times during which the patients are practicing the techniques. Relaxation techniques depend on meditation and related physical practices to produce physiological changes opposite to those evoked by stress. Biofeedback equipment detects changes in heart rate, blood pressure, muscle tension, and other physiological phenomena, the awareness of which will help the individual voluntarily alter body processes that were once thought not to be under voluntary control. Schwartz has shown, for example, that people can be taught to alter both their heart rates and blood pressures.

Benson and Schwartz think that such methods should be useful as adjuncts to, but not as replacements for, drug therapy. One of the big problems with therapy for high blood pressure, however, is motivating the patient to continue the treatment; it remains to be seen whether patients will comply with the requirements of biofeedback or relaxation methods any more rigorously than they comply with drug therapies.

Alvin P. Shapiro of the University of Pittsburgh School of Medicine is one of the many investigators holding out for the view that the preponderance of evidence favors a connection between stress and chronic high blood pressure, even though the exact role of stress is hard to determine. He emphasizes that investigators generally agree that disturbances in any of several interacting systems or organs, such as the endocrine system, the brain, and the kidneys, could result in chronically elevated blood pressures. The problem is that, as the number of factors involved increases, it becomes more difficult to sort out the role played by each. Considering how difficult it is to pinpoint the roles of the physiological factors, which are easy to quantify compared to stress, it is not at all surprising that the results of some studies designed to test the stress hypothesis have been unsatisfactory.

6

EXERCISE AND HEART DISEASE
Equivocal Evidence

Most people who embark on exercise programs do so because they believe regular exercise is good for them. They are encouraged in this belief by physicians and by what are often evangelical articles in the popular press. Medical scientists generally agree that, at the very least, exercise promotes weight control and a general sense of well-being. But many people believe that exercise does something more — that it prevents them from developing heart disease. Unfortunately, this supposed benefit has yet to be firmly established and what evidence there is for it is equivocal.

If exercise has not been proved to prevent heart disease, why do so many authorities encourage people to exercise to prevent heart disease? The answer seems to be that even some of the methodologically flawed studies have yielded results that exercise proselytizers can interpret in favor of their theory. For example, it is clear that physically active people have less heart disease and are more likely to survive heart attacks than those who are not active. What is not clear is that exercise is the sole factor offering this protection to the active people. If one is willing to assume that reducing risk factors for heart disease actually reduces risk (a premise not yet proven), then additional evidence that may be interpreted in favor of exercise has been reported.

The story of researchers' attempts to determine whether exercise prevents heart disease reads like a tale of woe. For more than 20 years, investigators have actively searched for a relation between exercise and heart disease. They have compared incidences of heart disease among people who exercise regularly (such as longshoremen and mail carriers) to incidences among people with more sedentary jobs. They have asked whether college athletes and marathon runners are less likely to suffer heart disease than the rest of the population. They have initiated clinical trials to see whether men who are seemingly disease-free will have fewer heart attacks if they participate in an exercise program and whether men who have already had heart attacks will live longer if they exercise. But despite this monumental effort, every study has been flawed.

One of the biggest problems with research on exercise and heart disease is self-selection of subjects. That is, those people who exercise regularly, or even those who can be persuaded to exercise regularly, are often different from the rest of the population. They are less likely to smoke or to be obese, for example. Thus they do not in any sense constitute a representative cross section of the population.

This problem of self-selection creeps into nearly all retrospective studies of exercise and heart disease. For example, it is often cited as contaminating results of comparisons of heart disease rates among active and sedentary workers. Results from one of the first studies of this kind were reported in 1953, and numerous studies have been carried out since — all with the same drawback. In this initial study, J. N. Morris and his associates at the London School of Hygiene and Public Health compared the rates of heart disease of conductors and drivers in the London Transport System. The conductors, who walked up and down the aisles collecting fares, were more active than the drivers, and the conductors had only 70 percent as much heart disease as the drivers. (These incidences were corrected for age.)

The problem, however, is that men were not randomly allocated to jobs as conductors or drivers. The leaner men in this population chose or were assigned to be conductors, whereas the heavier men chose or were assigned to be drivers. As Morris himself later pointed out, drivers, on entering employment, were of a greater average girth for a given height than conductors.

Self-selection also doomed attempts to conduct a randomized, controlled clinical trial to see whether exercise prevents heart disease. Such a trial was recommended in the early 1960s by a committee convened by the Heart Disease Control Program of the Public Health Service, and a pilot study to see whether a large-scale trial would be feasible was subsequently initiated. Three universities (the University of Minnesota, the University of Wisconsin, and Pennsylvania State University) participated in the pilot study. The study involved a total of 385 men between the ages of 40 and 59 who were randomly assigned to treatment and control groups. Those in the treatment group participated in three 1-hour exercise sessions each week.

Unfortunately, this pilot study failed because so many participants dropped out of the exercise group. By the end of 6 months, the drop-out rate was about 50 percent. Thus the study would not suffice to determine heart disease incidences among those who remained in the exercise group because of the problem of self-selection — that is, people apparently do not drop out randomly.

Some valuable information was nonetheless obtained from the pilot study. The investigators learned that people generally cannot be coerced or persuaded to exercise regularly over long periods of time. In fact, even a desire to exercise may not be enough since quite a few dropped out of the exercise group because of injuries. The investigators sadly concluded that "relatively high intensity physical activity is impractical in large scale trials of primary prevention of heart disease."

Because of these admitted failures to demonstrate that exercise prevents heart disease, exercise advocates have been unable to use either retrospective studies or clinical trials to clinch their argument. The retrospective studies are especially equivocal because much of the "positive" evidence is balanced by negative evidence from similar studies. For example, although many studies showed that those whose jobs require physical activity are less likely to develop heart disease than those with more sedentary jobs, a number of similar studies failed to demonstrate such a relationship. And although some investigators found that people such as college athletes and marathon runners have lower incidences of heart disease than the population at large, others have not obtained such results. It remains possible, of course, that the negative studies involved populations in which the differences in activity between the active and inactive groups were too small to be reflected in the incidences of heart disease. Considering this problem, Arthur Leon of the University of Minnesota says it is surprising and encouraging that so many of these population studies did show any effects of exercise.

Many promotors of exercise supplement their claims that exercise prevents heart disease by citing studies other than these retrospective ones. For example, they cite results from the prospective Framingham Study and results of studies indicating that exercise might reduce risk factors for heart disease.

As part of the Framingham Study, which was directed by William Kannel, the physical activity of 207 men was assessed by a method which was described as "admittedly crude." Kannel and his associates prepared a physical activity index for each man, based on the amount of time he said he devoted each day to various kinds of physical activity, such as sitting, walking, standing, and more vigorous forms of activity. The Framingham investigators followed the 207 men for 10 years, and at the end of that time they found that the more active men had lower incidences of heart disease than the more sedentary men, even when established risk factors (such as smoking, high blood pressure, and high concentrations of blood cholesterol) were taken into account.

The Framingham investigators were extremely cautious in interpreting their results. They concluded, "What is really surprising, then, is that we are able to demonstrate the hypothesized relationship between physical activity and CHD at all, not that it is only of marginal statistical significance, and that it is only observed for men and is statistically significant only when all ages are considered jointly. Still, one might wish for better data and firmer conclusions."

Recently, Ralph Paffenberger and his associates at the University of California at Berkeley reported evidence that men (aged 35 to 74) who exercise vigorously may have fewer heart attacks. These investigators sent questionnaires to Harvard alumni asking them to describe their customary physical activity and state of health. The men who reported expending at least 2000 calories per week through exercise had 64 percent fewer heart attacks over a 6- to 10-year period than the more sedentary men. Of course, the usual objection that the healthier men are those who will exercise still holds, but this study has been highly touted as evidence that strenuous exercise may protect against heart disease.

Indirect evidence that exercise might prevent heart disease comes from studies of the effects of exercise on the heart and the rest of the body. These studies indicate that exercise might, at the very least, reduce risk factors for heart disease. (These results might be questioned, however, since none of the studies were prospective. And the pilot study for a clinical trial on exercise and heart disease did not show any effect of exercise on risk factors.)

Arthur Leon and Henry Blackburn of the University of Minnesota report that numerous investigators, in retrospective studies of athletes, sedentary people, and animals, have documented such beneficial effects of exercise. Regular exercise seems to result in a reduction of the heart rate and blood pressure, greater cardiovascular efficiency in delivering oxygen and nutrients to body tissues, and reduction in the heart's oxygen requirements for a given amount of work. Blood clots less easily (which may reduce the risk of coronary thrombosis), and people lose fat and gain muscle tissue. Cells become more sensitive to insulin. (Diabetes, in which cells are relatively insensitive to insulin, is a risk factor for heart disease.) In addition, a greater proportion of blood lipids are carried by high-density lipoproteins – a condition thought to be associated with protection from heart disease.

The relation between exercise and risk factors for heart disease was further investigated by Kenneth Cooper and his associates at the Institute for Aerobics Research in Dallas and reported in 1976. These researchers examined 3000 men (average age 44.6 years) for heart disease risk factors and to determine cardiovascular fitness (which they measured with a treadmill and electrocardiogram monitors). They found that the more physically fit men had statistically significantly lower concentrations of serum cholesterol, triglycerides, and glucose and that they had lower blood pressures. Of course it is possible, if not likely, that the more physically fit men were able to exercise regularly because they were healthier. That is, the reduced risk factors may be a precondition of their fitness rather than a result of it.

Nonetheless, the investigators at the Institute for Aerobics Research are encouraged by their initial results and are now initiating a long-term study to see whether men who exercise regularly at the institute will, over a period of years, reduce their risk factors for heart disease. They expect to enroll 5000 men in the study and are counting on a 50 percent drop-out rate over 3 years. They say that they expect such a relatively low drop-out rate because the enthusiasm for and belief in exercise at the institute is infectious.

Even if exercise alone does not reduce risk factors, there is some evidence that people who embark on and adhere to exercise programs may change their life-styles in such a way as to reduce their risk factors. The net effect, whatever the cause, of this reduction in risk factors may then protect against heart disease. For example, William

Haskell of Stanford University finds that middle-aged Stanford faculty members who take up jogging also tend to cut down on their cigarette smoking and change their eating habits.

Although exercise or changes in life-style associated with exercise may reduce risk factors for heart disease, this does not necessarily mean that it reduces the incidence of heart disease. For example, many investigators, including Robert Levy, director of the NHLBI, believe that heart disease develops slowly over a period of 20 to 50 years. One commonly held opinion is that heart disease occurs in response to constant and prolonged injury to arteries by such factors as high blood pressure, substances in cigarette smoke, and high concentrations of serum cholesterol. If so, a middle-aged man who suddenly takes up exercise may be doing so too late to prevent himself from developing heart disease, even if he does reduce his risk factors.

Some more definitive answers to the question of whether exercise prevents heart disease may be forthcoming from current studies on both risk-factor reduction and effect of exercise on life-span of heart attack patients. The NHLBI is currently conducting two large-scale clinical trials to answer the question of whether reducing risk factors reduces incidences of heart disease. But some argue that even these trials will not resolve this issue, and, in any event, the results of these trials will not be in for several years.

The argument that exercise may prevent heart disease by reducing risk factors becomes even less satisfying in the case of the post-heart attack patient. As Basil Rifkind of the NHLBI points out, risk factors become far less important after a person has had a heart attack. What is important then is the amount of injury done to the person's heart. It may be argued that exercise can also help the heart attack patient by making the damaged heart more efficient. Whether this is so is now under active investigation.

Six clinical centers are participating in the National Exercise and Heart Disease Project, a clinical trial that involves a total of 651 heart attack patients, randomly assigned to an exercise group and a control group. The participants are all highly motivated, according to Patrick Gorman of George Washington University, which should reduce the drop-out rate. However, the participants' motivation may cause another problem. John Maughten of the State University of New York at Buffalo reports that some members of the control group are moving into the exercise group. This could again cause problems in the interpretation of results.

Although there have been several previous attempts to study the effects of exercise on heart attack patients, most of these investigations have also been methodologically flawed. The only reported results from a randomized controlled trial are from a study of patients in Göteborg, Sweden, conducted by L. Wilhelmen, H. Sanne, and D. Elmfeldt of the University of Göteborg. These investigators randomly assigned 128 patients to exercise and control groups. However, 25 percent of these patients were found to have injuries that precluded their exercising. After 1 year, 40 percent of the exercise group had dropped out; after 4 years, 75 percent had dropped out. But the mortality rate among those who adhered to the exercise program for 4 years was only a third of that of either the drop-outs or the control group (both of whom had similar mortality rates). It is possible, of course, that those who continued to exercise were simply healthier to start with than those who dropped out.

Blackburn points out that there are disadvantages of intensive exercises after a heart attack. For example, patients may place themselves in increased danger of cardiac arrest. According to Blackburn, physicians often lack the interest, experience, and facilities to supervise exercise programs. Medical researchers generally agree that patients must be selected and evaluated by stress tests before they are put on an exercise schedule. But, says Blackburn, this test is not only limited by availability and cost, it is also not always a good indicator of who will benefit or suffer from exercise. He concludes that most heart attack patients should be encouraged to gradually increase their physical activities, but that vigorous exercise should be reserved for the patient qualified by stress tests, accustomed to regular and strenuous exercise, and who greatly desires to resume exercising.

Currently available evidence, then, on the role of exercise in preventing heart disease or rehabilitating heart attack patients is equivocal. Those who want to believe in exercise can find encouraging hints that it may be beneficial. Those who do not can argue that exercise may not do much good. As Michael Pollock of Mt. Sinai Hospital in Milwaukee puts it, "The evidence is on the fence. What you conclude depends on whether or not you're a believer in exercise." And, given the difficulties of obtaining conclusive rather than suggestive evidence, this dilemma may remain unsolved for some time.

III

Etiology

7

ETIOLOGY OF
HEART DISEASE
Current Research Trends

To find out what causes heart disease, medical scientists must first uncover the cause or causes of atherosclerosis. Angina pectoris and most heart attacks are the result of the buildup of atherosclerotic plaques in the coronary arteries. These deposits of arterial smooth muscle cells, lipids, and calcium partially or completely block the arteries, producing rough, irregular surfaces that may trigger the formation of blood clots. Blood flow to a portion of the heart muscle is thus reduced, and it may be cut off entirely. Atherosclerosis contributes to the death of some 640,000 heart attack victims every year. When the plaques form in the arteries of the brain, they may lead to strokes, which claim an annual toll of an additional 200,000 lives.

As yet investigators have not had much success in pinpointing the cause or causes of atherosclerosis. They agree, however, that the abnormal proliferation of the smooth muscle cells of the arterial lining appears to be a key element in the process. Consequently, they are expending a great deal of effort to find out why this happens. Two major theories currently dominate the research. One of them is an old theory that is gaining new adherents. It maintains that plaques form as result of injury to the innermost lining of the arteries, with subsequent exposure of the underlying muscle cells to substances from which they are normally shielded. Some of these substances may then stimulate the cells to divide, thus thickening the arterial wall and narrowing the inner diameter of the artery at various points.

The second theory, the monoclonal hypothesis, holds that each plaque is a clone; that is, that all the cells in it are derived from the division of a single parent cell. In this view, a plaque is a kind of tumor that arises as a result of a process akin to that causing cancerous tumors, although the plaque tumor is benign in the sense that its growth does not overwhelm and kill the host directly.

Proponents of both theories have suggested that the known risk factors for coronary heart disease — cigarette smoking, hypertension, and elevated concentrations of blood cholesterol — could enhance the development of plaques in ways consistent with both theories. Cigarette smoke, for example, might injure arterial walls. Or it could trigger the abnormal division of smooth muscle cells in the arterial lining — a not unreasonable idea since the smoke is known to carry chemicals that cause cells to become cancerous.

Hypertension, in which the pressure of blood in the arteries is higher than normal, is another risk factor that may help trigger the atherosclerotic process by putting undue strain on arterial linings and damaging them. Of course, hypertension is not just a risk factor for atherosclerosis. Since it can lead to heart and kidney failure and to stroke, it is a serious problem in its own right. Investigators now realize that hypertension is a complex of diseases rather than a single pathological entity. They have implicated several hormonal and neural mechanisms that might lead to chronic elevations in blood pressure. The problem is that, as more factors are involved, it becomes increasingly difficult to determine the exact role of each factor.

The role of cholesterol in the genesis of atherosclerotic plaques also continues to puzzle researchers. This lipid is a prominent component of the plaques, and most investigators are convinced that high concentrations of cholesterol in blood do contribute to plaque formation. The manner in which this happens is uncertain, but there is recent evidence, at least in experimental animals, that chronically elevated blood cholesterol concentrations may contribute to arterial damage.

But results from biochemical and epidemiological studies now indicate that simple measurement of the total concentration of cholesterol in blood may not be an adequate indicator of an individual's risk of having a heart attack. Biochemical studies have shown that cholesterol is transported in the blood in complexes with proteins and other lipids. There are four major classes of these lipoprotein complexes, each with a different function. Of particular interest here are the low-density lipoproteins (LDL), which carry cholesterol to the peripheral tissues where it is used, and the high-density lipoproteins (HDL), which act as "garbage trucks" that pick up cholesterol not used by the tissues and carry it to the liver where it can be broken down or excreted into the intestines. Epidemiological evidence suggests that high concentrations of LDL increase the risk of having a heart attack, whereas high concentrations of HDL decrease that risk, a possibility consistent with their known physiological functions.

It is too early to tell whether it will ever be possible to deliberately alter the concentrations of HDL and LDL to decrease an individual's risk of having a heart attack. Most attempts to influence blood cholesterol concentrations in the hopes of reducing the heart disease toll have focused on the use of cholesterol-lowering diets or drugs. Diet, especially, is often promoted to the public as a way of avoiding heart attacks, even though there is virtually no evidence that this will in fact save lives. The general feeling among members of the medical profession is that a low-cholesterol, low-fat diet will at least not hurt anyone — and it may be of benefit.

There are a few investigators, however, who think that general recommendations of dietary changes are premature. One of them, Edward Ahrens of Rockefeller University, thinks that a low-cholesterol diet may lower the blood cholesterol concentrations of some — but by no means all — individuals. Ahrens points out that the amount of cholesterol in the diet is just one factor that influences the concentration of this compound in blood and other tissues. In addition, the amount actually absorbed, the amount broken down or excreted, and the amount synthesized in the body must all be considered (especially since most cells can readily synthesize cholesterol).

Ahrens is investigating what happens when individuals ingest cholesterol and has found marked variations in the way their bodies handle it. Some respond by decreasing cholesterol synthesis sufficiently to compensate for the amount ingested; these persons experience no changes in their blood and tissue cholesterol concentrations. In contrast, some individuals cannot adequately compensate for ingested cholesterol by decreasing its production. But even in these individuals, there are significant differences in the fate of the increased cholesterol burden. In some, the plasma concentrations increase markedly. In others, the plasma concentrations remain unchanged whereas the amount stored in their other tissues increases greatly.

Ahrens says the people whose regulatory mechanisms do not compensate for dietary intake might benefit from a cholesterol-lowering regimen, but the others probably will not. He is now looking for a simple method of identifying those who might benefit.

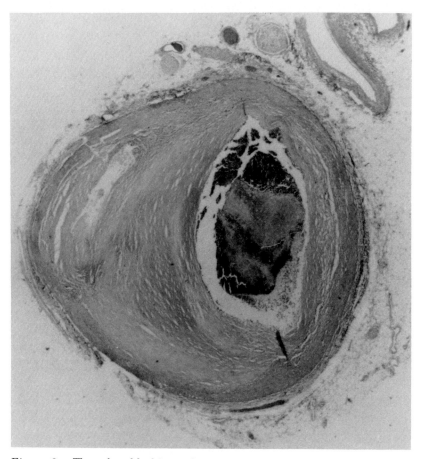

Figure 8. Thrombus blocking a human coronary artery that was already narrowed by an atherosclerotic plaque. The gray region is the plaque, which has almost filled the interior of the artery. The remaining open area has been totally occluded by the thrombus, which consists of white blood cells and platelets (the light region in the center of the photograph) and red blood cells (the dark area). [Source: Earl P. Benditt, University of Washington School of Medicine; reprinted with the permission of *Scientific American*]

Ahrens has been highly critical of the design of many of the epidemiological studies done or now under way that aim to study the effect of lowering blood cholesterol on the incidence of heart attacks. He says that they have failed to account for individual differences in the ways the subjects handle cholesterol. None of the studies done thus far have shown that lowering blood concentrations of cholesterol will prevent heart attacks, and Ahrens suggests that those in progress may also fail to do so. He fears that any benefits of the regimens being tested may go undetected if they help only a small percentage of the subjects.

Another component of the blood that has been implicated in the development of atherosclerotic plaques is the platelets, small disk-like cells needed for blood clotting. Some investigators think that platelets release factors that stimulate smooth muscle cell division and subsequent plaque formation. But no matter how the plaques form, both they and the platelets often cooperate in causing heart attacks because plaques may serve as initiation sites for thrombus formation. A thrombus is a type of clot composed mainly of clumped platelets, and a heart attack occurs if a thrombus forms in the coronary arteries (Figure 8). Investigators have recently determined that platelet aggregation, and presumably thrombus formation, is regulated by the balance between the opposing actions of two powerful chemicals. One, a prostaglandin produced in blood vessel linings, blocks aggregation; the other, a thromboxane produced by the platelets themselves, stimulates aggregation. The discovery of these chemical regulators has aroused a great deal of interest because of the possibility that it may lead to the design of new drugs that prevent or reverse thrombus formation.

In the past few years scientists have garnered a number of clues about the etiology of coronary heart disease from basic research. Nevertheless, translation of that information into lives saved is still in the future.

8

ATHEROSCLEROTIC PLAQUES
Competing Theories Guide Research

Atherosclerosis is frustrating to study and treat. The disease has no symptoms in its early stages, and since there is not yet an adequate noninvasive way to detect this disease, people generally do not know that they have it until they suffer a heart attack or stroke. At that point, no one can tell the victims why they, in particular, have developed atherosclerosis, or what they could have done to prevent it.

A major problem in understanding the etiology of atherosclerosis is that, like cancer, it seems to be a disease of many causes. Cigarette smoking, high blood pressure, high concentrations of blood lipids and cholesterol, excessive intake of animal proteins, various genetic disorders, and numerous other factors have all been linked to the development of this disease in susceptible individuals. This multiplicity of possible causes has stimulated investigators to look for some sort of common denominator—initial events in the genesis of atherosclerotic plaques that could be set in motion by any of these agents. The hope is that an understanding of how atherosclerotic plaques form will lead to new ways to prevent or reverse their development.

From examinations of human atherosclerotic plaques (Figure 9) and from studies of plaques in animals, researchers have come to agree that plaques consist primarily of arterial smooth muscle cells. These cells presumably proliferate and migrate from the middle layer to the inner layer of the arterial wall; as the plaques form, various substances such as connective tissue proteins and lipids accumulate.

Since the proliferation of smooth muscle cells seems to be central to the formation of plaques, investigators believe that an understanding of why and how plaques originate will come when they can determine what causes arterial smooth muscle cells to proliferate. To this end, they are, for the most part, examining the ramifications of two hypotheses.

The first hypothesis is an old one whose recent widespread support is based mainly on studies of lesions of animal arteries. It

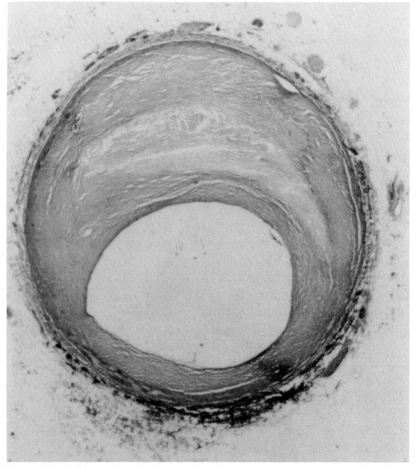

Figure 9.   Atherosclerotic plaque in a human coronary artery, enlarged 15 diameters. [Source: Earl P. Benditt, University of Washington School of Medicine; reprinted with the permission of *Scientific American*]

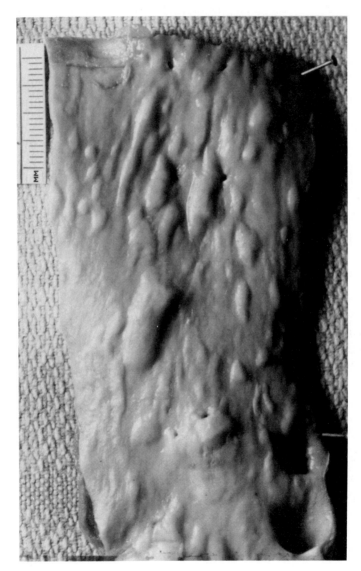

Figure 10. Atherosclerotic inner surface of a human aorta, enlarged about 1½ times. The plaques are seen as discrete lumps. [Source: Earl P. Benditt, University of Washington School of Medicine; reprinted with the permission of *Scientific American*]

states that plaques form in response to frequently recurring injuries to arterial walls. The competing hypothesis, which was first proposed about 3 years ago, states that plaques are benign tumors, each of which is formed by the progeny of a single cell that lost control of its growth. The two hypotheses lead to different predictions of how atherosclerosis can be prevented or controlled.

Proponents of the response-to-injury hypothesis point out that almost any kind of chronic damage to animal arteries leads to the development of lesions resembling human atherosclerotic plaques. In a variety of experimental animals, both direct mechanical injury and injuries stemming from antigen-antibody complexes, from applications of the amino acid homocysteine, and from high concentration of blood lipids have all produced arterial lesions. By analogy, supporters of this hypothesis suggest that humans can suffer arterial injuries from high blood pressure, antibodies to or carbon monoxide from cigarette smoke, high concentrations of blood lipids and cholesterol, and numerous other conditions.

By observing the genesis of lesions produced by injuries to arterial walls of animals (Figure 10), investigators have begun to piece together a sequence of events that is common to lesion formation in all animal species studied. They propose and have some evidence that the same sequence of events occurs when humans develop atherosclerotic plaques.

The first event in the development of lesions in animals is injury to the arterial endothelium, which is a thin layer of cells that coats the inner walls of arteries and controls the passage of large molecules in the blood through to the inner layers of the arterial wall. Once this barrier is disrupted, substances that normally are screened out by the endothelium can reach smooth muscle cells. For example, plasma lipoproteins, which are believed to supply lipids to the developing plaques, can then more easily contact smooth muscle cells. At the same time, platelets adhere to the newly exposed tissue, aggregate, and release substances that may stimulate cell proliferation. Subsequently, smooth muscle cells, which are normally present mainly in the middle layer of the artery, begin to proliferate and migrate to the inner layer where the injury occurred.

The proliferation of smooth muscle cells is surrounded by large quantities of connective tissue proteins and other macromolecules. As Russell Ross and his associates at the University of Washington School of Medicine have shown, arterial smooth muscle cells secrete these substances both in vivo and in vitro. Their accumulation is presumed to occur concomitantly with the multiplication of the smooth muscle cells. Supporters of the response-to-injury hypothesis claim that the resulting lesions in animals appear to be identical to lesions in humans that are considered to be precursors of athero- sclerotic plaques.

Several groups of investigators, including Ross, Sean Moore of McMaster University, and their associates, found that smooth muscle cells of injured animal arteries continue to proliferate and accumu- late connective tissue and lipids if the injuries are sustained or repeated. The lesions then resemble advanced atherosclerotic plaques in humans. Lesions in animals regress and eventually disappear if the injuries are not repeated, which leads many researchers to believe that repeated injury may be necessary for atherosclerosis to develop.

The central question that arises from this research is, Why do smooth muscle cells proliferate when the arterial endothelium is injured? In recent years, it has been suggested that the answer may lie in the responses of smooth muscle cells to various substances in the blood. One such substance seems to be present in the blood of people or animals with elevated concentrations of blood lipids. Robert Wissler, Katti Fischer-Dzoga, and their colleagues at the University of Chicago find that low-density lipoproteins (which carry cholesterol) from the blood of monkeys with hypercholesterolemia cause arterial smooth muscle cells to proliferate in tissue culture. No other fraction of serum from these monkeys produces this effect; neither do the low- density lipoproteins from monkeys with normal serum cholesterol concentrations produce this effect.

Other substances in the blood that may cause smooth muscle cells to proliferate are those released from platelets that aggregate at the site of injury to arterial walls. Ross and his colleagues report that a growth-stimulating factor is released from platelets when blood clots. When quiescent smooth muscle cells from monkey arteries are grown in tissue culture, this factor causes them to divide. When these cells are grown in the presence of cell-free serum, the cells remain in a resting state and maintain their original density. The addition of a protein released from platelets stimulates these cells to synthesize DNA and divide. R. Bruce Rutherford of the University of Washington School of Medicine and Ross found that, within 48 to 60 hours after they add the platelet protein, the number of cells doubles. These investigators point out that arterial smooth muscle cells are normally exposed only to filtrates of plasma, since the endothelium prevents the entry of platelets and other constituents of whole blood.

If a factor released from platelets is necessary in order for lesions to form, it should be possible to prevent the lesions after endothelial injury by preventing platelets from releasing this factor. Recently, several groups of investigators demonstrated that this can be done.

Moore, Robert Friedman of McMaster University, and their associates injured rabbit aortas by placing catheters so that they repeatedly hit the arterial walls. This injury causes fibrous plaques to develop. When the investigators treated the animals with antibodies to rabbit platelets, the lesions did not form. Similarly, Michael Stemerman, of Beth Israel Hospital in Boston, and his associates injured rabbit arteries with a catheter to which a balloon was attached. They inserted the catheter, inflated the balloon, and rubbed off endothelial cells with the balloon. Plaques normally occurred at the sites where the cells were rubbed off. After these investigators destroyed most of the rabbits' platelets with antibodies, they found that plaques no longer formed in response to the injury.

A different kind of injury was studied and its atherogenic effects prevented by Lawrence Harker, also at the University of Washington School of Medicine, Ross, and their associates. They continuously infused homocysteine into the bloodstreams of baboons for 3 months. Harker and Ross found that, as a result, the animals lost 10 percent of their arterial endothelial cells and developed lesions. Another group of baboons was given both homocysteine and the drug dipyridamole, which inhibits platelet functions and prevents the release of factors from platelets. These animals lost endothelial cells but did not develop lesions.

Platelets may be associated with the genesis of human atherosclerotic plaques as well as plaques in animals. The admittedly preliminary evidence is based on measurements in humans of platelet survival times, which indicate how long platelets circulate in the blood before breaking down. Platelet survival times are expected to decrease when platelets accumulate and break down at the site of arterial injury. For example, Harker, Ross, and their associates reported that platelet survival times are decreased 50 percent in baboons infused with homocysteine.

In addition to studying baboons, Ross, Harker, and their associates measured platelet survival times of patients with homocystinuria – an inborn error of metabolism that causes people to have large amounts of homocysteine in their plasma. These people typically die of atherosclerosis before they reach 30 years of age. The investigators found that a group of patients with this disease had platelet survival times that were 50 percent lower than those of controls.

Ross, Harker, and their associates further found that they were able to treat their homocystinuric patients so as to increase their platelet survival times. Some of the patients responded to the vitamin pyridoxine by producing less homocysteine, and they were treated with that vitamin. The rest were given dipyridamole. All of the treated patients subsequently had normal platelet survival times.

The results obtained by Harker and Ross were recently questioned by Joseph Schulman, S. Harvey Mudd, and their associates at the National Institutes of Health (NIH). They also measured platelet survival times in a group of patients with homocystinuria and found them to be normal.

Mudd explains that the results of the study of the NIH group do not necessarily contradict those of Harker and Ross. The patients studied by the NIH group were less severely affected by homocystinuria than the patients of Harker and Ross and presumably had less extensive arterial injuries. Measurements of platelet survival times are not particularly sensitive, and severe injuries to the arteries might be required before decreased platelet survival could be detected. It also remains possible (some say likely) that platelet factors are not solely responsible for the proliferation of smooth muscle cells and that normal platelet survival times do not necessarily indicate a lack of arterial damage and plaque formation. Conversely, shortened platelet survival times may not necessarily indicate that atherosclerotic lesions are progressing.

Stemerman and his associates recently obtained evidence that other factors may diminish the effects of platelet substances on the proliferation of smooth muscle cells in injured rabbit arteries. They find that after an artery is injured, smooth muscle cells of the resulting lesion begin to regress about 16 weeks after the initial injury. Yet these smooth muscle cells still have platelets attached to them. Healing begins when endothelial cells start to grow back over the lesions – a process that takes far longer than 16 weeks to be completed. Smooth muscle cells covered by new endothelial cells regress more rapidly than those not covered, according to Stemerman and his colleagues. Thus, the endothelium may be filtering out substances that stimulate, to some extent, the growth of smooth muscle cells. Stemerman points out, however, that the fact that smooth muscle cells regress while exposed to platelets indicates either that the cells can control their response to factors released from platelets or that other substances are involved in the stimulation of smooth muscle cell proliferation.

One factor that may be necessary to sustain smooth muscle cell proliferation is an elevated concentration of low-density lipoproteins in the blood. Wissler and his associates, among others, find that, in monkeys and swine with hypercholesterolemia, advanced atherosclerotic plaques shrink substantially when the animals' serum cholesterol concentrations are returned to normal. As the plaques shrink, the excess proliferation of arterial smooth muscle cells ceases.

Despite its widespread support among investigators, the response-to-injury hypothesis is based mainly on studies of animals. A major obstacle to extending findings from animal studies to humans is that initial events in human atherosclerosis are nearly impossible to identify. Human lesions are generally seen only at death or on the removal of an artery, and in neither case can the temporal development of the lesions be followed. Some investigators object to the response-to-injury hypothesis by saying that lesions of injured animal arteries are not necessarily comparable to human atherosclerotic plaques. There is disagreement about the validity of this objection among investigators. Proponents of the hypothesis that plaques are benign tumors—the monoclonal hypothesis—avoid this criticism since evidence supporting this hypothesis comes from studies of human plaques.

Earl Benditt and John Benditt of the University of Washington School of Medicine advanced the monoclonal hypothesis on the basis of an analysis of human plaques obtained at autopsies. Their analysis relies on a method that had been used previously to support the contention that benign uterine tumors made up of smooth muscle cells are derived from single cells. This method is based on the generally accepted belief that only one of the two X chromosomes in a given cell of a female expresses its genes and that the particular X chromosome in a cell that is active is decided at random during embryo development. All progeny of a particular cell express genes from the same X chromosome as their parent, but neighboring cells are often derived from different parent cells and thus often express genes from different X chromosomes.

One particular gene carried on X chromosomes codes for the enzyme glucose-6-phosphate dehydrogenase (G6PD). This enzyme can occur in two distinguishable forms, and black females tend to be heterozygous for the gene. Thus cells from black females who are heterozygotes will synthesize, at random, one or the other form of G6PD.

The Benditts examined atherosclerotic plaques from four black females and found that most cells collected from a single plaque expressed one or the other form of G6PD, but not both. They interpret this to mean that each plaque was generated by progeny of a single cell. In contrast, they found that cells from samples of artery walls adjacent to the plaques tended to produce both forms of G6PD.

In the 3 years since the Benditts advanced the monoclonal hypothesis, their results have been confirmed by other groups of researchers. Various investigators have published speculations as to how this hypothesis could be further tested and how previous results could be interpreted in light of it. Wissler, for example, believes that investigators should address the question of whether the arterial cells that seem to proliferate so readily when exposed to plasma lipoproteins are transformed cells. Ross points out that transformed arterial smooth muscle cells may not be affected by the same growth stimulants, such as factors released from platelets, as are normal arterial smooth muscle cells grown in tissue culture. Thus, in vitro studies of growth stimulants of smooth muscle cells may have to be reexamined.

Earl Benditt suggests that the meaning of proposed risk factors for atherosclerosis should be assessed in light of the monoclonal hypothesis. For example, cigarette smoking may be associated with this disease because cigarette smoke contains mutagens. And plasma lipoproteins may carry fat-soluble mutagens to arteries where these mutagens may pass through the arterial endothelium and contact smooth muscle cells. Benditt points out that diets high in fat have been associated with the development of various cancers, such as breast cancer, as well as atherosclerosis. He proposes that such diets may cause both cancers and plaques by similar mechanisms.

Although other investigators have confirmed the Benditts' results, several groups have recently raised objections to their interpretation. Philip Fialkow of the University of Washington, for example, points out that there is some evidence that plaques develop in layers. A group of cells may proliferate, then most die, and a few remaining cells proliferate again. If this is the case, a plaque could end up with cells of a single enzyme phenotype even though the plaque originated from many cells. Similarly, George Martin and his associates at the University of Washington School of Medicine argue that the Benditts' data do not necessarily indicate that plaques are formed by mutated or transformed cells. After studying a variety of cell lines, they discovered that cells that divide rapidly enjoy a selective advantage. Thus progeny of a single cell might take over a plaque that had a multicellular origin.

Somewhat different evidence against the monoclonal hypothesis is reported by Wilbur Thomas and his associates at Albany Medical College. These investigators found that plaques in swine are not monoclonal. They radioactively labelled the normal arterial tissue and induced lesions by feeding the animals diets high in cholesterol. If each lesion were formed from a single cell, the radioactivity of each lesion should be substantially less than the radioactivity of the surrounding cells of the artery. This did not occur. Instead the radioactivity of each lesion was not sufficiently diluted for it to be derived from one rather than many cells.

Thomas admits that the lesions in swine may not be analogous to those of humans, but he still maintains that the evidence advanced by the Benditts is not sufficient to support the monoclonal hypothesis. Despite these arguments against the monoclonal hypothesis, no one has yet succeeded in ruling it out. It, like the response-to-injury hypothesis, continues to have both supporters and detractors. Both hypotheses continue to suggest new experiments whose results, many believe, will narrow the range of possible causes of and ways to prevent atherosclerosis.

9

ATHEROSCLEROSIS
The Cholesterol Connection

Nobody doubts that cholesterol is a major component of athero-sclerotic lesions. That has been known for more than 100 years. The major questions that investigators have been trying to resolve concern the route by which cholesterol gets into the lesions, its role in their initiation and development, and — most important — whether lesion formation can be prevented or reversed with a consequent savings of some of the 900,000 lives lost every year to atherosclerotic disease in the United States alone.

Investigators have been using three approaches in their attempts to pin down the role played by cholesterol in the etiology of athero-sclerosis. One involves epidemiological or statistical studies. These have shown a correlation between high concentrations of blood cholesterol and an increased risk of having a heart attack, which may occur as a result of the formation of atherosclerotic lesions in the arteries that supply blood to the heart muscle. But the epidemio-logical studies have been criticized for a variety of reasons, and not all investigators think that the correlation is adequate proof of a causative relationship.

Another way to get at the problem involves studying the bio-chemistry of cholesterol in both normal and disease states. And the third approach encompasses studies designed to show whether low-ering the concentration of cholesterol in the blood by means of diet, drugs, or surgery will interfere with the progression of atherosclero-sis and actually prevent heart attacks.

The biochemical studies have resulted in a better understanding of how cholesterol is transported in the body and how its synthesis and utilization are controlled. Information of this kind may eventually lead to an unraveling of the mechanisms underlying the formation of atherosclerotic plaques and thus permit intervention to block the process. For example, high concentrations of one form of blood cholesterol apparently favor plaque formation. Investigators have made considerable progress in determining how the blood concentrations of this material are regulated.

Since cholesterol is a sterol (a steroid bearing an alcohol group; Figure 11), it is practically insoluble in water, and virtually all of the material in the blood is carried in the form of lipoproteins. These complexes of proteins with lipids are constructed with the charged or polar molecules, the proteins, for example, on the surface. The nonpolar molecules, such as triglycerides (esters of glycerol and three long-chain fatty acids) and esters of cholesterol, are on the inside. Seventy percent of the cholesterol in lipoproteins is present as esters. The free or nonesterified cholesterol is on the surface of the lipoproteins.

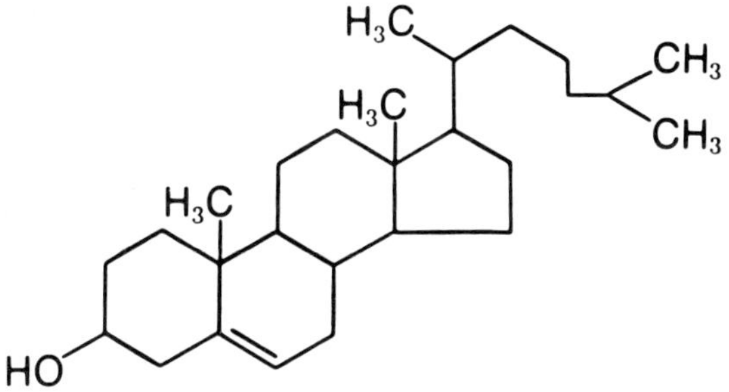

Figure 11.   Structure of cholesterol.

There are four main types of lipoproteins, which are classified according to their size and density. These are the chylomicrons, the very-low-density lipoproteins (VLDL), the low-density lipoproteins (LDL), and the high-density lipoproteins (HDL). Recently, attention has focused on the LDL, which are known to carry most of the cholesterol found in blood, as playing a key role in both the development of atherosclerotic lesions and in the regulation of cholesterol metabolism in cells other than liver cells. Much of the interest stems from the work of Michael Brown and Joseph Goldstein of the University of Texas Health Science Center at Dallas.

These investigators have evidence that human fibroblasts and certain other kinds of cells normally contain specific receptors for LDL, and that interaction of the lipoprotein with the receptors is a necessary first step before the degradation of LDL and the suppression of cholesterol synthesis can occur in the cells. If these two events are prevented, then large quantities of the cholesterol-bearing LDL may accumulate in the bloodstream. This is apparently what happens to persons with the genetic disease called familial hypercholesteremia. According to Brown and Goldstein, fibroblasts from these individuals lack receptors with the capacity to bind LDL.

Persons who inherit two copies of the gene that transmits this disease have concentrations of plasma cholesterol that may exceed 800 milligrams per 100 milliliters—roughly four times the normal value. They develop symptoms of atherosclerosis at a very early age and often die of heart attacks before their 20th birthday. Individuals who inherit one copy of the gene have plasma cholesterol concentrations that are about twice the normal value; they, too, develop symptoms of atherosclerosis prematurely but usually not before they are 30 years old.

However, only a small fraction—about 20 percent, according to some estimates—of persons with high blood concentrations of LDL actually have typical familial hypercholesteremia. The condition of most is the result of a poorly understood combination of hereditary and environmental factors. Nevertheless, the single-gene form of familial hypercholesteremia afflicts about one person in 500. And the fact that a single genetic defect results in both high concentrations of LDL in the blood and also severe atherosclerotic disease strengthens the case that blood cholesterol, most of which is carried in the LDL, is causally involved in atherogenesis.

Most, if not all, of the cells of the body have the capacity to synthesize cholesterol, a substance essential as a building block for cell membranes and also as a precursor for the synthesis of other steroids, including the bile acids and a number of hormones. Liver cells are especially active in synthesizing cholesterol, but synthesis is suppressed when the intake of dietary cholesterol is high. According to Marvin Siperstein of the University of Texas Southwestern Medical School, the dietary cholesterol acts by suppressing the synthesis of a key regulatory enzyme (3-hydroxy-3-methylglutaryl coenzyme A reductase) needed for cholesterol synthesis.

The results of John Bailey at George Washington University Medical School and George Rothblat at the Wistar Institute implied that a similar feedback inhibition was operating in peripheral cells. They observed that removal of cholesterol from the medium in which cultured mammalian fibroblasts are incubated enhances synthesis of the sterol by the cells. Brown and Goldstein then showed that the LDL suppress cholesterol synthesis by cultured human fibroblasts and that binding of the lipoprotein to the specific receptors on the fibroblast surface is a necessary first step toward the suppression.

According to the investigators, fibroblasts from patients with two genes for familial hypercholesteremia either have no receptors for LDL or else have defective receptors that bind LDL very poorly. They have observed both situations in the cultured cells. Fibroblasts from persons with one defective gene have half the normal number of functional receptors.

Brown and Goldstein suggest that, following binding of LDL to the receptors of normal cells, the membrane invaginates to form vesicles containing LDL inside the cell (Figure 12). With Richard Anderson, also at the University of Texas, they have shown that LDL labeled with ferritin, a protein that contains a large quantity of iron and can thus be seen in electron micrographs, binds to the membrane of normal cells at certain areas that are indented and have fuzzy coats. Other investigators have suggested that these areas are the sites where formation of the internal vesicles is initiated. Although cells from patients with familial hypercholesteremia have the indented areas, they do not bind the ferritin-labeled LDL the way normal cells do.

The next step is the merger of the vesicles with the lysosomes (membranous sacs containing enzymes that break down a variety of biological molecules). The enzymes digest the protein components of LDL and split the cholesterol esters with the release of free cholesterol, which is the form used by cells to synthesize membranes. In addition, the liberated cholesterol has three important regulatory roles. It reduces cholesterol synthesis by suppressing the key regulatory enzyme; it activates another enzyme (cholesterol acyltransferase), which catalyzes the formation of new cholesterol esters for storage; and it suppresses the synthesis of the LDL receptor and thus prevents accumulation of too much cholesterol by the cell.

Support for the role of the lysosome in this scheme comes from experiments in which Brown and Goldstein showed that cells deficient in a lysosomal enzyme that splits cholesterol esters can accumulate LDL in the lysosomes but that the esters are hydrolyzed at a reduced rate. Thus, the release of free cholesterol is delayed, as are the regulatory events.

However, if these cells or the cells lacking the receptors are supplied with free cholesterol in a form that can penetrate the membrane, they will respond to the sterol in the normal manner. That is, the enzyme regulating cholesterol synthesis will be sup-

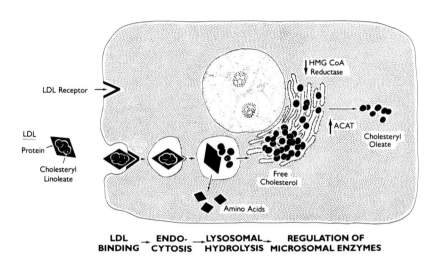

LDL → ENDO- → LYSOSOMAL → REGULATION OF
BINDING CYTOSIS HYDROLYSIS MICROSOMAL ENZYMES

Figure 12. Scheme showing the uptake of low-density lipoproteins (LDL) by the cell and their subsequent fate. The LDL are composed of protein and cholesterol esters, mainly the ester cholesteryl linoleate. The LDL bind to their receptors, and the membrane bearing the receptors bulges inward to form vesicles inside the cell. (This process is called endocytosis.) After the vesicles fuse with lysosomes, the lysosomal enzymes break the protein portion of the LDL down to amino acids and split the cholesterol esters, producing free cholesterol. Free cholesterol affects the activities of two microsomal enzymes. (Microsomes are composed of interior membranes of cells with their attached ribosomes; they are the site of synthesis of many complex biochemical molecules.) It inhibits the enzyme designated HMG CoA reductase and consequently decreases the synthesis of more cholesterol. It also stimulates the enzyme designated ACAT and thus enhances the synthesis of another cholesterol ester called cholesteryl oleate. Thirdly, the free cholesterol decreases the formation of LDL receptors by the cell and thus prevents more cholesterol than is needed from entering the cell. [Source: Joseph L. Goldstein and Michael Brown of the University of Texas Health Science Center at Dallas. Reprinted with the permission of *Science*]

pressed and the one reesterifying the sterol will be activated. According to Andrew Kandutsch of the Jackson Laboratory, certain oxygenated derivatives of cholesterol are even more effective than the parent compound in producing these responses in both normal cells and those from individuals with familial hypercholesteremia. This could point the way to more effective methods for lowering elevated blood cholesterol concentrations than are now available.

Brown and Goldstein think that the effects of LDL, acting through the receptor, could explain the low rate of cholesterol synthesis normally seen in many cell types in vivo. On the other hand, lack of functional receptors could contribute to elevated LDL concentrations in the blood in two ways. Peripheral cells would be unable to take up and metabolize LDL adequately. In addition, the enzyme regulating cholesterol synthesis would not be suppressed and the cells would continue to produce the sterol in spite of the high plasma concentrations.

Recent epidemiological studies also support the concept that high concentrations of LDL may contribute to the development of atherosclerosis and coronary artery disease. William Kannel, director of the prospective Framingham Study, says that their data indicate that, as the concentration of plasma LDL increases, the risk of having a heart attack also increases. On the other hand, persons with high concentrations of HDL have fewer heart attacks than persons with low concentrations, according to Kannel and William Castelli, also of Framingham. The effects of the two lipoproteins on the risk of coronary heart disease appear to be independent of one another. This result, and those from other investigations, imply that HDL may somehow protect against the development of atherosclerotic lesions.

These findings are consistent with the physiological roles postulated for LDL and HDL in cholesterol transport. Investigators* think

---

* Many investigators have contributed to the elucidation of lipoprotein structure and the pathways by which lipoproteins and the cholesterol contained in them are transported and utilized. They include Donald Fredrickson, now director of the National Institutes of Health; John Glomset of the University of Washington; Antonio Gotto of Baylor Medical School; Richard Havel of the University of California Medical School in San Francisco; Robert Levy, currently director of the National Heart, Lung, and Blood Institute; Angelo Scanu of the University of Chicago; Bernard and Virgie Shore of the Lawrence Livermore Laboratory of the University of California; Olga and Yechezkel Stein of Hebrew University–Hadassah Medical School in Jerusalem; and Donald Zilversmit of Cornell University.

that lipoproteins do not just function to solubilize lipids, but that the proteins on the surfaces of the particles carry information that specifies the tissues to which the different classes of lipids are to be delivered. The proteins would do this by recognizing and interacting with receptors on the appropriate cells or by serving as cofactors that are necessary for the action of the enzymes involved in shuttling cholesterol and other lipids from tissue to tissue.

The pathways by which the different lipoproteins are formed, interconverted, and used are complicated, but the view emerging from a large number of studies is that the LDL carry cholesterol, whether obtained from the diet or synthesized in the body, to the peripheral tissues where it is used. Goldstein and Brown think that the bulk of the LDL may be degraded in tissues other than the liver. This hypothesis is supported by findings from the laboratory of Daniel Steinberg of the University of California at San Diego. He showed that removal of the livers of swine did not slow the degradation of cholesterol by the animals and may even have increased it.

On the other hand, the HDL appear to transport cholesterol from the peripheral tissues to the liver. From here it may be excreted into the intestinal tract either as cholesterol or after conversion to the bile acids. Alternatively, it can be incorporated into LDL or VLDL and recycled to the peripheral tissues. But the HDL may provide a route for removal of cholesterol from the tissues and, possibly, for diminishing the likelihood of its ending up in atherosclerotic plaques.

The way in which high concentrations of blood cholesterol contribute to the production of atherosclerotic lesions is still unclear. One hypothesis, proposed by Russell Ross and Lawrence Harker of the University of Washington School of Medicine, is that chronic elevation of the sterol concentration leads to local injury to the inner lining of the arterial wall. When the investigators increased the blood cholesterol concentration of monkeys by feeding the animals a diet high in the sterol, about 7 percent of the inner surface of their major arteries suffered damage. The arteries of control monkeys remained intact.

Several investigators have suggested that arterial injury is a major factor in the formation of atherosclerotic plaques. The idea is that this would expose the smooth muscle cells beneath the injury to blood constituents that stimulate the local proliferation of the smooth muscle cells. Not everyone agrees that arterial injury is the cause of the proliferation, but most investigators think that abnormal growth of the smooth muscle cells is a key factor in the formation of atherosclerotic plaques. Moreover, evidence from a number of laboratories, including that of Robert Wissler at the University of Chicago, indicates that the LDL promote the division of arterial smooth muscle cells, possibly by providing lipids for cell membrane formation. Thus, high concentrations of cholesterol-containing LDL may be involved in the initiation of lesion formation as a consequence of injury to the arterial lining, and the lipoproteins may also contribute directly to lesion progression.

Atherosclerotic plaques contain large deposits of cholesterol. Several factors, acting alone or in combination, could be contributing to the accumulation. The cholesterol could be taken up directly from the blood; elevated concentrations of LDL might facilitate this uptake. The mechanisms by which arterial smooth muscle cells use the cholesterol might be deficient. Or the cells might be synthesizing the sterol in larger than normal quantities. There is evidence for all three of these possibilities.

Smooth muscle cells from human arteries take up large quantities of LDL and VLDL, at least in culture, according to Edwin Bierman and his colleagues at the University of Washington School of Medicine. They take up lesser quantities of HDL. These results contrast with those the investigators obtained with cultured smooth muscle cells from rat arteries. The latter cells take up more HDL than LDL or VLDL. Bierman points out that the rats are very resistant to the development of atherosclerosis, whereas humans readily develop the condition. He suggests that the ease with which a species develops atherosclerosis may be related to this difference in lipoprotein uptake. According to Bierman, the characteristics of LDL binding and uptake by the cultured cells are consistent with the presence on the arterial cells of receptors similar to those observed by Brown and Goldstein on cultured human fibroblasts.

Bierman has also found that lowering the oxygen content of the atmosphere above the cultured cells decreases the breakdown of the protein portion of the LDL and causes the protein to accumulate in the cells. Since degradation of LDL proteins is part of the normal sequence for breakdown of the LDL, Bierman thinks that oxygen deficiency could promote accumulation of LDL and accelerate the formation of the lipid-laden cells seen in atherosclerotic plaques. He has hypothesized that this may be one way that cigarette smoking, which is a known risk factor for atherosclerosis, contributes to plaque formation. The carbon monoxide inhaled by smokers replaces some of the oxygen that would otherwise be carried by hemoglobin and consequently lowers the arterial oxygen pressure.

Once the lipoproteins have been taken up by the aortic smooth muscle cells, the lysosomes may play an important role in determining whether or not atherosclerotic lesions develop, according to Christian de Duve of the Rockefeller University and the University of Louvain in Belgium. The lysosomes contain the enzyme (cholesteryl esterase) that splits the cholesterol esters that form the bulk of the LDL cholesterol; the splitting occurs after the lysosomes fuse with the vesicles carrying the LDL. A prominent feature of the lesions are the foamy cells which are thought to be formed from smooth muscle cells that have accumulated large quantities of cholesterol and have consequently lost their characteristic structure. Since cholesterol must be released from its esters in order to be used by the cells or transported out of them, de Duve thinks that, if the lysosomes of arterial smooth muscle cells were deficient in cholesteryl esterase, cholesterol esters would accumulate and the foamy cells might result.

De Duve has evidence that this is what occurs when rabbits are fed a high-cholesterol diet and consequently develop atherosclerosis. He and his colleagues have found that the lysosomes of the aortic smooth muscle cells of cholesterol-fed rabbits are much less dense than those of normal animals. This is what would happen if the lysosomes were accumulating lipids of low density. The Rockefeller investigators have also determined that the activity of the cholesteryl esterase in rabbit lysosomes is very low. De Duve hypothesizes that this activity is adequate to split the cholesterol esters ingested by rabbits on their normal vegetarian diet, which contains little of the sterol; however, when the animals are fed high-cholesterol diets, the enzyme can no longer handle the esters taken up by the cell and thus they accumulate.

The LDL appear to inhibit cholesterol synthesis by aortic smooth muscle cells in culture just as they do in fibroblasts. Brown and Goldstein have observed the inhibition in smooth muscle cells from human aortas, and Steinberg has observed it in swine cells. Steinberg points out that at the concentrations of LDL thought to occur in the fluid bathing aortic smooth muscle cells in vivo, normal cells should be synthesizing very little cholesterol and most of the cholesterol accumulating in atherosclerotic lesions ought to come from the blood.

The situation could be quite different in cells from patients with familial hypercholesteremia if they resemble fibroblasts in their lack of feedback inhibition by LDL. Here, cholesterol synthesis by the aortic smooth muscle cells could make an important contribution to the sterol accumulating in the arterial lesions of the patients.

Although the preponderance of the evidence favors the hypothesis that cholesterol, especially that carried by the LDL, is somehow involved in atherogenesis, the big question remains to be answered. That is, will lowering the concentration of cholesterol in the blood prevent or reverse the process of plaque formation and save the lives of persons who would otherwise have died of heart attacks or strokes?

Animal studies do indicate that the lesions will regress when the blood cholesterol is lowered. Many of the species used, however, differ markedly from the human in physiology and diet. There is always the possibility that experimental atherosclerosis in animals like the rabbit is not a good model for the human variety.

Recently, however, encouraging results have been obtained with swine and nonhuman primates, both of which are physiologically similar to the human. For example, Assad Daoud and his colleagues at Albany Medical College observed that advanced atherosclerotic lesions in the arteries of swine would regress if the animals were put on a low-cholesterol diet. The investigators induced the lesions in the first place by a combination of mechanically injuring the arterial lining and feeding a high-cholesterol diet.

Monkeys can also be made to develop advanced atherosclerosis if they are fed appropriate diets. And their lesions will regress if the animals are switched back to a low-cholesterol diet, according to Mark Armstrong of the University of Iowa. In a recent experiment, Wissler and his colleagues fed rhesus monkeys a diet containing large quantities of coconut fat, butterfat, and cholesterol for 18 months. Those animals killed at the end of this time all had severe atherosclerotic lesions in the coronary arteries. The remaining monkeys were divided into three groups. One continued to receive the high-fat, high-cholesterol diet; the other two received either a low-cholesterol diet or a low-cholesterol diet plus a drug thought to prevent atherosclerosis in monkeys. According to Wissler, the frequency and severity of the lesions of the monkeys on the low-cholesterol diets were 30 to 50 percent lower than those of the control animals. The drug produced some additional improvement in the appearance of the arteries of the monkeys receiving it.

Although researchers consider the results of the animal investigations to be encouraging, the only way to tell whether the same is true for humans is by studying humans. In at least one such study, it was not. The Coronary Drug Project, sponsored by the National Heart, Lung, and Blood Institute and completed late in 1974, was designed to determine whether the use of drugs that lower blood cholesterol would decrease the incidence of heart attacks in men who had already had at least one. It turned out that men taking the drugs had as many heart attacks as those receiving a placebo.

However, investigators think that these negative results do not necessarily disprove the value of lowering blood cholesterol concentrations. The average decrease in the blood cholesterol seen in the study was modest at best—less than 10 percent—and possibly was too late to do any good. By the time a heart attack occurs the atherosclerotic process may be well advanced.

Another approach is to study individuals whose atherosclerosis is not so far advanced but who are at risk of having a heart attack. The NHLBI is currently sponsoring two major prospective trials involving men thought to be at risk. The first of these, the Lipid Research Clinic Primary Prevention Trial, aims at determining whether otherwise healthy men with high blood cholesterol concentrations can decrease their chances of having a heart attack by lowering their cholesterol concentrations. The second trial, the Multiple Risk Factor Intervention Trial, includes men who have one or more of the three risk factors, high concentrations of blood cholesterol, high blood pressure, and cigarette smoking, considered most predictive of the likelihood of having a heart attack. Attempts are being made to reduce or eliminate all of the risk factors and to determine whether there is a reduction of heart attacks. However, it will be at least 5 years before the results of either of these studies are available.

Meanwhile, there are two techniques that investigators think may permit them to obtain results faster than by long-term prospective studies. One involves using surgery to produce much greater decreases in blood cholesterol than the 10 to 20 percent decreases usually achieved by diets or drugs. This might cause a more rapid regression of plaques. The other requires actual observation of the interiors of arteries to determine what, if any, changes occur as a result of a cholesterol-lowering regimen. Changes in the lesions should be detected earlier than altered incidence of heart attacks.

Henry Buchwald and his colleagues at the University of Minnesota Medical School have devised an operation, the partial ileal bypass, that reduces blood cholesterol concentrations by 30 to 60 percent. In the operation, the last third of the small intestine is disconnected from the intestinal tract to interfere with the absorption of cholesterol and the bile salts. The bile salts are needed to emulsify cholesterol and other lipids so that they can be absorbed. Most of the absorption of lipids and bile salts, which are recycled, occurs in the last third of the small intestine. Thus, after the surgery both the bile salts and cholesterol are excreted in the feces. Moreover, the liver continues to convert additional cholesterol to bile salts in order to replace those that have been lost. These, too, are excreted; this constitutes a further drain on the body's cholesterol. Buchwald says that the only side effects of the operation are diarrhea, which can be controlled with drugs, and a deficiency of vitamin B_{12}, which is also absorbed in the last third of the small intestine. This deficiency can be compensated for by injections. An advantage of the surgery is that the patients cannot cheat as they may do with diet or drugs.

More than 100 patients, most of whom have coronary heart disease and high blood cholesterol concentrations, have undergone the operation. Buchwald says that there is evidence that for some of them the condition of the coronary arteries has improved. He performed coronary angiograms on 22 patients before the surgery and then periodically thereafter for up to 3 years. Angiograms permit the visualization of arteries, here the coronary arteries, to see whether or not they have been blocked by atherosclerotic lesions. The atherosclerosis of 12 patients at least did not progress; that of three patients showed definite improvement; and that of two additional patients may have improved.

This was not a controlled study, but the NHLBI is now sponsoring a more extensive clinical trial, involving several clinical centers, to confirm that the surgical technique can cause improvement of atherosclerotic lesions in patients with coronary artery disease. The trial will ultimately include 1000 patients; 500 will undergo the surgery and 500 will be treated conventionally.

A sensitive technique for observing what is happening within the arteries before atherosclerotic lesions become large enough to actually block the vessels and cause symptoms could help to provide information about whether or not early lesions will regress. David Blankenhorn and his colleagues at the University of Southern

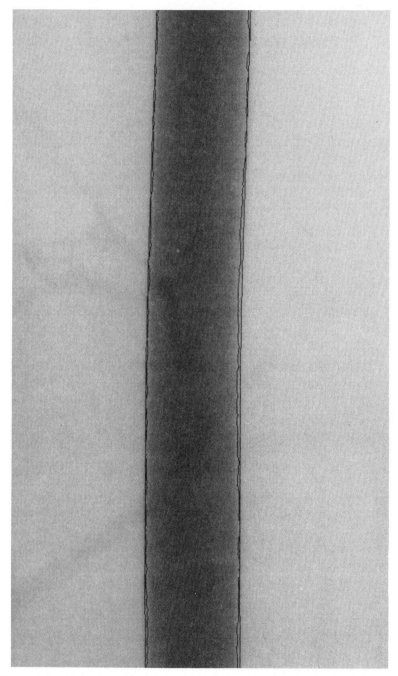

Figure 13. Computer-reconstructed images of human femoral arteries. In the photographs the inner lines show the actual edges of the arteries as determined by computer analysis of angiograms; the smooth outer lines represent what should be the normal boundaries of the arteries as calculated

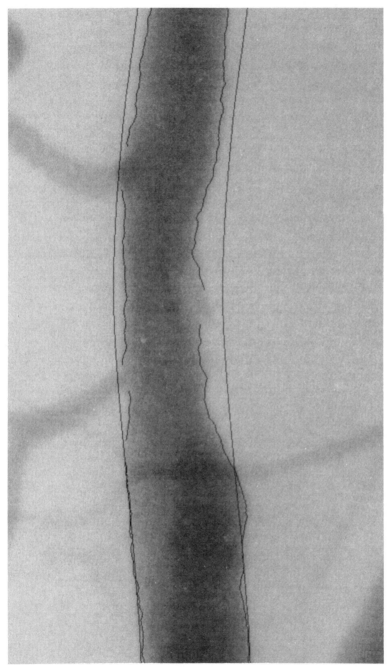

by the computer. (Facing page) Image of a femoral artery with little or no atherosclerotic disease. (Above) Image of an artery severely deformed by advanced atherosclerosis. [Source: David Blankenhorn of the University of Southern California]

California have applied computer technology originally developed for the analysis of photographic images taken by spacecraft to the analysis of angiograms of the femoral artery of the thigh (Figure 13). With their technique they can visualize the plaques and determine whether they change in size over a period of time.

The investigators have performed a series of angiograms on 25 men who have high concentrations of lipids, including cholesterol, in their blood. Before therapy to reduce the blood lipids and also high blood pressure, where required, the men all had moderately severe atherosclerosis of the femoral artery but did not yet have symptoms of obstruction. Blankenhorn is using a variety of drug and diet therapies on the men. After 13 months of treatment, nine of the 25 patients experienced regression of the lesions, whereas the lesions of 13 got worse and those of three did not change.

Blankenhorn says that the patients whose lesions regressed showed significant declines in blood cholesterol concentration; these decreases did not occur in individuals whose disease progressed. Statistical analysis of the data indicated that decreases in blood pressure made an independent contribution to the rate of change of the atherosclerosis, with a decrease favoring regression. Blankenhorn thinks that the changes in the femoral artery are representative of those that may occur in early lesions of the coronary arteries, but confirmation of this hypothesis will require the development of a similar technique for examining the coronary arteries.

10

BLOOD CLOTTING
The Role of the
Prostaglandins

The discovery late in 1976 of a new prostaglandin that appears to prevent formation of blood clots has begun a new chapter in the story of these potent regulatory chemicals. The recent discovery complements an earlier finding of a thromboxane (thromboxanes are close chemical relatives of the prostaglandins) that is extremely effective in causing blood platelets to clump and arteries to constrict, both effects that should promote blood clotting. Since the new prostaglandin has exactly opposing effects, the emerging picture is that the balance between the activities of the two agents may determine whether or not a clot will form.

The findings are of potentially great clinical significance because heart attacks and strokes are often caused by abnormal clot formation. Investigators hope that a better understanding of how the prostaglandins affect clot formation will lead to the development of new drugs that prevent clots. The structure of the prostaglandin has been determined, and it may be possible to synthesize a stable analog that mimics its action. Aspirin, an old drug that is now known to block prostaglandin synthesis, is already being tested in a clinical study sponsored by the National Heart, Lung, and Blood Institute to see whether it can protect against heart attacks.

Investigators have known for some time that the prostaglandins affect the aggregation of platelets in the test tube. Platelet clumping in response to blood vessel injury is one of the first steps in clot formation. However, it was difficult to work out the exact role played by the prostaglandins in the living animal. The body makes several prostaglandins, and some of them promote platelet aggregation, whereas others inhibit it. Investigators simply did not know enough about where and how the agents were synthesized and what controls the synthesis to determine which are physiologically important in regulating blood clotting.

A development that helped to clarify the situation — and that of prostaglandin biochemistry in general — was the discovery a few years ago of the prostaglandin endoperoxides. Then, in 1975, Mats Hamberg, Bengt Samuelsson, and their colleagues at the Karolinska Institutet in Stockholm identified the thromboxanes. Because both the endoperoxides and the thromboxanes are very unstable substances, they were hard to find and are hard to study.

The endoperoxides, now designated PGG_2 and PGH_2, are key intermediates in the synthesis of several prostaglandins and the thromboxanes (Figure 14). They are formed by the enzyme cyclooxygenase from arachidonic acid, a common fatty acid present in fats and other lipids. The enzyme is inhibited by aspirin and related compounds such as indomethacin, which thereby block the synthesis of all the prostaglandins and thromboxanes formed from PGG_2 and PGH_2.

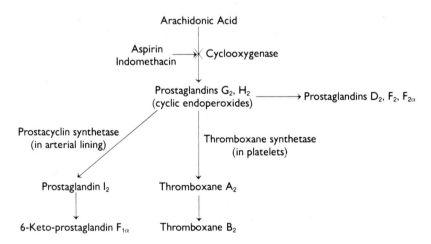

Figure 14. Scheme showing the major steps in the conversion of arachidonic acid to the prostaglandins and thromboxanes. Prostaglandin I_2, which inhibits platelet clumping and arterial constriction, is formed by an enzyme in blood vessel linings. The enzyme that synthesizes thromboxane A_2, which has the opposite effects, is located in platelets. The breakdown products, 6-keto-prostaglandin $F_{1\alpha}$ and thromboxane B_2, have little or no biological activity.

Although platelets clump when they are exposed to endoperoxides, the Karolinska group thinks that much, and possibly all, of this effect can be attributed to the fact that endoperoxides serve as a source of the thromboxane called TXA_2. Samuelsson and Hamberg have shown that TXA_2 is an extremely potent aggregator of platelets. In addition, the investigators have evidence that the agent is identical with "rabbit aorta contracting substance" originally described by John Vane and Priscilla Piper, then at the Royal College of Surgeons in London. Both materials contract rabbit aortas, have similar half-lives, and are formed in platelets from endoperoxides.

The enzyme that synthesizes TXA_2 (thromboxane synthetase) has been identified in platelets by investigators from Vane's laboratory at Wellcome Research Laboratories in Beckenham, England, working in collaboration with Hamberg and Samuelsson. The Wellcome group included Philip Needleman, who was then on sabbatical from Washington University School of Medicine, and Salvador Moncada. The enzyme is located in the platelet microsomes, small vesicles composed of fragments of interior cell membranes.

While examining other types of tissues to see if they too contain the enzyme, Moncada and Vane found that microsomes prepared from pig and rabbit aortas do not form TXA_2; instead, they contain an enzyme that converts the endoperoxides to a previously unknown, highly unstable prostaglandin that prevents or reverses platelet aggregation and relaxes several kinds of blood vessels. The investigators at first named this material prostaglandin X. The name was changed to prostacyclin after structural analysis showed that it contains a ring not found in other prostaglandins (Figure 15).

The structure was determined last fall by a group of investigators at the Upjohn Company under the direction of Roy Johnson. They proved the structure of the new prostaglandin by synthesizing it, the classic means by which chemists establish the structure of a compound. The Upjohn group, in collaboration with Moncada and Vane, then showed that the properties of the synthetic material were the same as those of natural prostacyclin. The full chemical name of the material is (5Z)-9-deoxy-6,9α-epoxy-Δ^5-prostaglandin $F_{1\alpha}$. Most recently, the compound has been designated PGI_2, following the alphabetical nomenclature scheme applied to previously described prostaglandins.

The investigators could predict the structure of prostacyclin because those of its immediate precursor, PGG_2, and of its breakdown product, 6-keto-prostaglandin $F_{1\alpha}$, were known. The latter substance had previously been discovered in stomach tissue by Cecil Pace-Asciak of the Hospital for Sick Children in Toronto. He showed that this compound was the major stable product formed from the endoperoxides and postulated that the compound called PGI_2 was the immediate precursor of the stable keto derivative. Pace-Asciak was also the first investigator to isolate PGI_2, although he did not study its biological activity. He isolated the material in 1970 but at that time did not have enough of it to determine the complete structure. (The configuration of the groups around one of the double bonds was unknown.)

Moncada and Vane have shown that PGI_2 is synthesized in human arteries and veins and in bovine coronary arteries in addition to pig and rabbit aortas. They say that the enzyme that generates PGI_2 is located in the innermost lining of the blood vessels. According to these investigators, PGI_2 is the predominant product formed from the endoperoxides in blood vessel linings, whereas in platelets the endoperoxides are converted into TXA_2 and other prostaglandins but not into PGI_2.

Moncada and Vane postulate that the formation in platelets and blood vessel linings of agents with opposing effects provides a mechanism for the normal control of blood clotting and suggests an

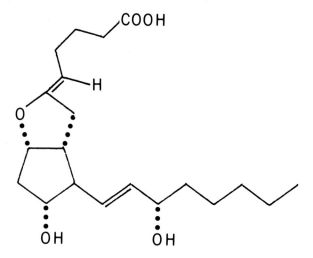

Figure 15.   The structure of PGI_2 or prostacyclin.

explanation for the genesis of atherosclerotic plaques. Normally, platelets do not stick to the inner linings of arteries and veins even though they are known to adhere easily to many other kinds of surfaces. The investigators think that when platelets come in contact with the linings, they release endoperoxides. These are then converted to PGI_2 (which prevents the platelets from aggregating and forming a clot) by the enzyme in blood vessel linings. However, where blood vessels are damaged there would be a lack of the PGI_2-synthesizing enzyme (prostacyclin synthetase) and clot formation could occur.

Many investigators think that destruction of the inner lining of arteries is one of the initial steps in the formation of atherosclerotic plaques. Moreover, platelets are present in the plaques and possibly promote formation of the lesions. Thus, in the view of Moncada and Vane, loss of the cells containing prostacyclin synthetase may be a major contributor to the atherosclerotic process. Furthermore, the lesion sites would themselves lack the enzyme, a situation that would encourage further clot formation and increase the danger that the artery would become blocked. These investigators have also shown that a lipid hydroperoxide effectively inhibits the activity of prostacyclin synthetase. Moncada and Vane speculate that the presence of lipid peroxides in atherosclerotic plaques might help explain the increased clotting problems of patients with atherosclerosis.

Although blockage of a coronary or cerebral artery by the atherosclerotic plaques or a blood clot may cause, respectively, a heart attack or a stroke, arterial constriction can also temporarily reduce the flow of blood and deprive tissue of needed oxygen. The effects of TXA_2 on the contraction of arterial smooth muscle could make an additional contribution to the disease process, whereas the opposing effect of PGI_2 may help to protect against restriction of blood flow.

John Oates, Earl Ellis, and their colleagues at Vanderbilt University have demonstrated that when human platelets aggregate in the presence of thrombin (a natural promoter of clotting), they release a labile substance that causes the contraction of porcine coronary arteries. They identified the substance as TXA_2 and hypothesized that platelets, if they aggregate in regions where the lining of the coronary arteries is damaged, could release the agent. Consequent constriction of the arteries could then play a causative role in heart attacks and in the transient blood flow restriction to the heart muscles in angina pectoris.

In contrast, Needleman and his colleagues have evidence that coronary arteries release a substance that relaxes arterial smooth muscle. The investigators at first thought that it was PGE_1, an already known smooth muscle relaxer. Further studies ruled out that possibility by showing that arachidonic acid, which is not converted to PGE_1, relaxes preparations of coronary arteries. Indomethacin added with the arachidonic acid not only blocked the relaxing effect but also caused the arteries to contract. Needleman says that this result suggests that arachidonic acid was not active itself but had to be continuously converted to an unstable prostaglandin that causes the relaxation.

Although the investigators subsequently showed that the endoperoxide PGH_2 relaxes coronary artery muscle, they have evidence that the endoperoxide is converted to another labile compound that is much more potent. This material has all the characteristics of PGI_2. For example, Needleman and his colleagues find that bovine coronary arteries incubated with labeled arachidonic acid convert it to 6-keto-prostaglandin $F_{1\alpha}$, the stable breakdown product of PGI_2.

Needleman says that the coronary blood vessels produce PGI_2 when the heart is stimulated by the hormone bradykinin or when it is made oxygen-deficient as a result of the temporary obstruction of the coronary arteries. He thinks that by promoting dilation of the coronary arteries and increasing blood flow, PGI_2 may help to protect the heart muscle when the demand for oxygen is great, as in times of stress, or when blood flow to the organ is restricted.

Although most investigations of PGI_2 activity have been carried out in vitro, investigators are beginning to look at the effects of the agent in intact animals. For example, Peter Ramwell and his colleagues at Georgetown University Medical School and the Naval Medical Research Institute have found that PGI_2 injections into dogs and rhesus monkeys markedly reduce blood pressure. They think that the agent works by relaxing the smooth muscle of blood vessel walls. In monkeys it decreases the resistance to blood flow of the systemic circulatory system, an effect usually attributed to dilation of the small arteries.

The discovery of the role of TXA_2 and PGI_2 in blood clotting may make it possible to design more effective strategies for preventing heart attacks. Investigators do not expect that PGI_2 itself will be very useful in this regard because it is unstable, although it might be of some benefit if given by continuous intravenous injection to hospitalized patients. The agent both reverses and prevents aggregation of platelets and could help to dissolve clots that have already formed. But clinicians would no doubt prefer longer-acting agents. Chemists are already trying to synthesize stable analogs of PGI_2, as well as investigating another approach to preventing blood clotting, that of developing specific inhibitors of the enzyme that synthesizes TXA_2.

E. J. Corey and his colleagues at Harvard University have synthesized PGI_2 and four analogs that have been tested in in vitro systems by Ramwell. All the analogs inhibit the aggregation of human platelets induced by incubating them with adenosine diphosphate, but none are as potent as some of the natural prostaglandins. For example, PGE_1 is 20 times more effective in preventing platelet aggregation than the most active analog.

Although the effects of these analogs are not impressive, cardiovascular disease is such an important health problem that a large number of PGI_2 analogs will undoubtedly be synthesized and tested for their action on blood clotting. Upjohn chemists in particular are rumored to have already made some 200 compounds, and numerous other investigators are also actively working on similar syntheses.

One problem that they all will have to face is that most prostaglandins act on more than one system. Thus it is difficult to design an agent to affect only the desired target and have no unwanted side effects. For example, PGI_2 reduces blood pressure, and since the agent is found in tissues other than blood vessels, it may have additional unknown effects. Nevertheless, the high stakes make inevitable a large research effort to find a specific inhibitor of blood clotting.

Meanwhile the NHLBI has already started a clinical trial to determine whether aspirin, one of the oldest and most common drugs now in use, can save lives by preventing heart attacks. The trial, which is called "AMIS" for the Aspirin Myocardial Infarction Study, includes 4524 patients who have already suffered at least one heart attack. The NHLBI estimates that this prospective trial will cost a total of $17 million by the time it is completed. The experimental phase of AMIS will be finished in August of 1979.

Initial hopes for the outcome of AMIS were high. Aspirin is an inexpensive drug and is relatively safe, at least compared to other agents that may be used to treat heart attack victims. And the demonstration that it could prevent potentially fatal heart attacks would be of great benefit. However, the discovery that PGI_2 inhibits blood clotting and arterial contraction has led some investigators to question whether taking aspirin could prevent heart attacks.

The problem is that aspirin inhibits the first step of prostaglandin synthesis from arachidonic acid (Figure 14) and thus blocks the formation of PGI_2 as well as TXA_2, a potent promoter of blood clotting and arterial constriction. Most investigators agree that if, as seems likely, it is the balance between the activities of PGI_2 and TXA_2 that determines whether or not clotting will occur, the information is not now adequate to predict the effects of aspirin on the process.

The results of a half-dozen or so already completed studies have been mixed. Some indicated that aspirin might protect against heart attack. For example, some participants in the Coronary Drug Project, which was sponsored by the NHLBI and completed in 1975, took 1 gram of aspirin (the equivalent of about three standard aspirin tablets) every day. These patients appeared to have fewer heart attacks than the controls. Other studies, however, gave negative results. Vane has suggested that aspirin inhibition of both PGI_2 and TXA_2 synthesis may account for the lack of dramatic results. In any event, the anticlotting prostaglandin was discovered only after the completion of these trials and after recruitment for AMIS was completed in August 1976.

According to William Friedewald of the NHLBI, the institute decided to undertake AMIS because the inconclusive results of the earlier studies suggested the need for a trial that was well-designed, prospective, and double-blind (neither the patient nor the physician know who is getting aspirin and who placebo). He says that the discovery that aspirin inhibits TXA_2 synthesis, although not the rationale for the NHLBI study, did lend credence to the suggestion that aspirin might protect against heart attacks.

The participants in AMIS have been randomly divided into control and experimental groups. Those receiving aspirin take 1 gram of the drug every day. Friedewald says that the patients will be carefully watched for possible aspirin side effects, such as gastrointestinal bleeding and liver and kidney damage.

One criticism directed at AMIS — and at other large clinical trials being conducted by the NHLBI — is that such studies are very expensive; critics think that they drain off money that might be better spent on basic research. For example, Ramwell suggests that putting the money into a search for a specific inhibitor of the enzyme that synthesizes TXA_2 or for a stable compound that mimics the effects of PGI_2 might be more valuable in the long run. At the moment, however, no such agent is available. And as long as 10 years may be required to get Food and Drug Administration approval for use of a new drug in humans, whereas aspirin is already available as an over-the-counter drug.

Another argument that can be made in favor of a study to determine whether aspirin prevents heart attacks is that local effects in diseased coronary arteries may be different from those in normal blood vessels. Oates agrees that PGI_2 production may prevent clot formation in normal blood vessels, but he points out that diseased coronary arteries having severe atherosclerotic lesions may have few lining cells capable of producing the prostaglandin. Here the effects of TXA_2 release by platelets may well predominate and contribute to heart attacks and angina pectoris. Thus, inhibiting synthesis of the thromboxane might help persons with diseased arteries. Oates is beginning a trial to determine whether aspirin can benefit patients with unstable angina, a severe form of the condition in which individuals experience chest pain due to inadequate blood flow to the heart even when at rest.

A final question that has been raised about the AMIS trial concerns the dose used. Philip Majerus of Washington University School of Medicine says that recent results from his laboratory suggest that it may be too high. He and his colleagues have found that platelet cyclooxygenase is extremely sensitive to the drug; much less aspirin is needed to inhibit the platelet enzyme than the one from sheep seminal vesicles, for example. When the investigators gave aspirin to human volunteers, they found that a daily dose of as little as 180 milligrams produces 99 percent inhibition of the platelet enzyme. This is far less than the amount needed to achieve anti-inflammatory and analgesic effects. It is equivalent to about one-half of a standard aspirin tablet — or about one-sixth of the quantity taken by AMIS participants.

Majerus says that the results suggest that if the dose used in the aspirin trial is excessively high, it may at best be associated with more side effects than would be found with a low dose; at worst, it may inhibit cyclooxygenase in vessel linings in addition to that in platelets and thus prove ineffective. Majerus thinks that there may well be a role for aspirin in heart attack prevention but points out that "it would be irritating if we had to do the whole trial over again with a lower dose."

11

HYPERTENSION
A Complex Disease with Complex Causes

Hypertension, which afflicts 24 million people in the United States, is the most common of the chronic diseases. It is a major health problem because people with high blood pressure are more likely to have strokes, heart disease, or kidney failure than are people with lower blood pressure. Fortunately, when high blood pressure is lowered by appropriate therapy—and the therapy is effective in the vast majority of cases—the risk of heart or kidney failure and stroke falls along with it.

For the most part, however, finding the therapy to control a patient's high blood pressure is more of an art than a science. Physicians try various drugs or drug combinations until they hit on one that works. This is because 90 percent of the patients have what the medical profession calls "essential" hypertension. "Essential" means that no one knows what causes the condition. Medical researchers hope that current investigations into the mechanisms that regulate blood pressure will enable them to understand what causes chronic hypertension and provide a more rational basis for designing therapies for the condition.

One of the conclusions of the research is that hypertension is actually a complex of diseases in which different defects produce the same result—the elevated blood pressure. Therefore it is not surprising that drugs that work for some persons may not work for others who have different defects.

The idea that hypertension could have more than one cause was not unexpected. Although the blood pressure depends mainly on two factors—the resistance of the circulatory system to the flow of blood through it and the volume of fluid contained within the blood vessels—regulation of the two factors requires a complex set of interactions between the circulatory, nervous, endocrine, and excretory systems. A disturbance in any one could upset the balance required to maintain normal blood pressure.

For the past 10 to 15 years investigators have focused much of their attention on the role of renin, an enzyme produced by the kidney, in regulating blood pressure. Renin catalyzes the splitting of angiotensinogen, a protein found in blood, to form angiotensin I, a peptide containing ten amino acid residues. Another enzyme removes two of the residues from angiotensin I to yield angiotensin II (Figure 16). The heptapeptide angiotensin III is a third member of the angiotensin family.

The angiotensins act to increase blood pressure by influencing both peripheral resistance to blood flow and blood volume. At one time, all the actions were attributed to angiotensin II. Angiotensins I and III were thought to be physiologically inactive precursor and breakdown products, respectively, of the octapeptide. Recent evidence indicates that each angiotensin may be active, although in different ways.

Angiotensin II causes the constriction of the arterioles. These are small arteries that branch to form the capillaries, which are the smallest blood vessels and the sites where the blood exchanges nutrients and waste products with the tissues. The state of constriction or dilation of the arterioles is the most important determinant of the resistance to blood flow of the circulatory system and, therefore, of the amount of pressure required to force the blood through the circulatory system.

Stimulation of aldosterone secretion by the cortex or outer layer of the adrenal gland is a second consequence of angiotensin II formation. Aldosterone is a steroid hormone that acts on the kidney to increase retention of sodium ions and water. The resulting augmentation of the fluid content of the circulatory system elevates the blood pressure. Angiotensin II also acts directly on the kidney to increase sodium retention.

The third action of the angiotensins involves the nervous system. They stimulate the release of the neurotransmitter norepinephrine by the nerve terminals of the sympathetic nervous system and by the adrenal medulla (the inner portion of the adrenal gland), and potentiate the action of the norepinephrine. The sympathetic nervous system is the branch of the autonomic nervous system that helps the organism respond to stress. One of the effects of norepinephrine release is increased blood pressure caused by constriction of the arterioles.

A drop in the pressure of the blood flowing through the kidney is one stimulus of renin release. The normal signals that tell the kidney to stop releasing renin are an increase in blood pressure and angiotensin itself, which acts by a feedback mechanism to inhibit renin release. The result is that the pressure is not maintained above normal levels for long periods. But when these feedback mechanisms go awry, chronic hypertension may result.

The known causes of hypertension include kidney damage and a narrowing of the arteries leading into one or both kidneys, with the result that the arterial pressure always appears low to the kidney. These conditions may be dangerous since the pressure may be very high, but they can frequently be cured by removing the kidney or repairing the artery. Another known cause of hypertension is excess secretion of aldosterone, which may be due to the presence of a tumor

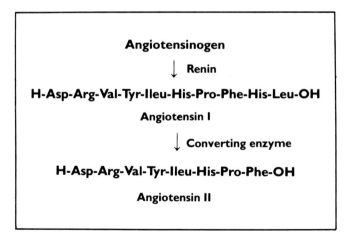

Angiotensinogen

↓ Renin

H-Asp-Arg-Val-Tyr-Ileu-His-Pro-Phe-His-Leu-OH

Angiotensin I

↓ Converting enzyme

H-Asp-Arg-Val-Tyr-Ileu-His-Pro-Phe-OH

Angiotensin II

Figure 16. Formation and structures of the angiotensins. Angiotensin I is produced by the action of the enzyme renin on angiotensinogen. The converting enzyme then removes the two amino acids from the right-hand end of angiotensin I to form angiotensin II. Angiotensin III is a heptapeptide containing the same amino acids as angiotensin II with the exception of the aspartic acid residue present on the left-hand end of the latter molecule.

of the adrenal cortex, for example. Again surgery will effect a cure of the hypertension. These causes account for only about 10 percent of all cases of hypertension.

At least some of the 90 percent of patients who have essential hypertension have elevated concentrations of renin in their blood even though they have no apparent sign of kidney damage. John Laragh and his colleagues, first at the Columbia-Presbyterian Medical Center and more recently at the Cornell University Medical Center in New York City, have been analyzing the amount of renin in the blood of hypertensive patients. The investigators find that 16 percent have high renin activity in the blood plasma and 27 percent have low activity. Renin values are normal in the remaining 57 percent. Laragh says that these differences show that hypertension is a heterogeneous disease in which not all patients present the same clinical picture. He thinks that classification according to plasma renin activity provides a guide to both the prognosis and therapy of a patient.

Laragh has found that patients with high plasma renin activity have the highest incidence of heart attacks, strokes, and kidney failure, whereas patients with low activity have lower risks of the serious consequences of high blood pressure. He thinks that the difference depends on whether increased vasoconstriction or increased blood volume is predominant in elevating a given patient's blood pressure.

In the first group, the problem would be vasoconstriction as a result of the activity of renin and the angiotensins. Although these patients also have high concentrations of aldosterone in their blood, many do not have increased blood volume because the hypertension, which was induced by the vasoconstriction, causes increased excretion of fluid; as a result, the plasma volume may actually be reduced and the blood viscosity increased. This combination of increased vasoconstriction and blood viscosity could put a great deal of stress on the blood vessels. Fortunately, therapy with the drug propranolol usually controls the blood pressure in these cases, possibly by decreasing renin secretion.

Laragh thinks that the condition of the second group is due mainly to an expanded arterial blood volume and that the increased pressure suppresses renin secretion. Thus, the organs and blood vessels of low-renin patients would be less subject to the extra stress imposed by renin vasoconstriction.

Among the possible causes of the expanded fluid volume would be decreased sodium excretion by the kidney or increased aldosterone secretion. Arthur Guyton and his colleagues at the University of Mississippi Medical Center have suggested that the kidneys of all hypertensive patients may be defective in their capacity to secrete sodium; at high blood pressures normal kidneys would secrete the ion in increased quantities and thus return the pressure to normal. In any event, Laragh thinks that diuretics, drugs that increase fluid excretion by the kidneys, are the best therapy for the low-renin patients.

The largest group of patients with essential hypertension are those with normal renin concentrations. These individuals have a risk of serious consequences almost as great as those with high renin activity. Even though their renin concentrations appear normal, Laragh thinks that they may actually be inappropriately high since the high pressures should suppress production of the enzyme. Also, in accord with Guyton's suggestion, the patients' kidneys may be defective in excreting salt, with the result that the blood volume is increased. Laragh hypothesizes that subtle defects in the kidney may be responsible for the initiation of the normal-renin hypertension. Some of these patients respond to diuretics alone and some to drugs that combat renin production; others require both.

Not everyone agrees with Laragh's hypothesis concerning the significance of blood renin concentrations in patients with hypertension. Some investigators say that their measurements of blood volume and other indicators of the condition of the cardiovascular system produce findings in conflict with those predicted by Laragh's theories. For example, they find that blood volume may be increased in patients with high plasma renin activity whereas Laragh suggests that it is decreased.

Regardless of the contribution renin makes to the development of chronic hypertension, many clinicians question whether adequate therapy requires time-consuming and expensive tests like those for measuring renin activity in blood. The Joint National Committee on Detection, Evaluation, and Treatment of High Blood Pressure has recently recommended an approach to therapy that does not use such tests but relies instead on a step-by-step testing of drugs to find the right combination to control an individual's blood pressure.

Accurate measurement of the renin activity can be difficult, because the results may be influenced by a variety of factors, including the salt intake of the patients. Another way to assess the contribution that elevated renin is making to a particular case of hypertension is the use of antagonists to angiotensin II (the production of angiotensin is determined by that of renin).

In order to produce its effects, angiotensin II must first combine with specific receptors on the target organs. Angiotensin antagonists are peptides that resemble the natural substance in that they bind to the receptors and prevent angiotensin from binding. The antagonists produce the same effects as the natural substance, but only when they are given in high concentrations; at low concentrations the antagonists block the action of angiotensin.

A number of investigators, including F. Merlin Bumpus of the Cleveland Clinic Foundation and Garland Marshall and Philip Needleman of Washington University School of Medicine, have synthesized angiotensin antagonists. The general approach involves replacement of one or more of the amino acids of angiotensin II with different amino acids. At present, the most commonly used antagonist is the octapeptide Saralasin that was the first synthesized by Donald Pals and his colleagues at the Norwich Pharmacal Company.

When Saralasin is injected intravenously into a patient with hypertension, the blood pressure falls to normal if the elevation is totally due to the activity of angiotensin and, thus, renin. If angiotensin makes no contribution to the increase, the blood pressure will not decrease. Or if the elevation in blood pressure is partly caused by angiotensin II, the drop will be proportional to the contribution made by the octapeptide.

This kind of information may be useful to the clinician in designing appropriate drug therapies. An inhibitor of renin release, for example, would be of little value for a patient whose hypertension is not caused by inappropriately high concentrations of renin. Several investigators, including Laragh, William Pettinger of the University of Texas Southwestern Medical School, and David Streeten of the Upstate Medical Center of the State University of New York, are using Saralasin in this manner.

Although the design of more effective therapeutic agents is one of the goals of the investigators synthesizing angiotensin antagonists, the antagonists now available can only be used on a limited scale. Because they are peptides, they must be administered by intravenous injection and even then they are rapidly degraded in the blood. But, in addition to their diagnostic applications, the current angiotensin antagonists are useful for studying the mechanisms of hypertension and also the mechanisms by which other drugs act. This latter kind of information should be useful in designing new drugs.

The observation that renin release or blood volume or both are abnormal in patients with hypertension does not explain what causes the abnormalities. For example, they may be in the kidney itself, as Guyton has suggested. The nervous system is another possible location of the origin of the aberrations. The interaction between angiotensin and the sympathetic nervous system, in which the hormone increases the release of sympathetic neurotransmitters such as norepinephrine and potentiates their effects on target organs, has been known for some time. But the central nervous system also plays a role in regulating blood pressure, and this too appears to involve the renin-angiotensin system.

In an early experiment in 1961, Joseph Buckley of the University of Houston showed that angiotensin II could act through the central nervous system to increase blood pressure in the dog. Since then a number of investigators have confirmed this observation in additional species. Buckley, for example, showed that injection of small amounts of angiotensin II into the brain of the cat caused rapid and significant increases in blood pressure. The effect could be blocked either by cutting through the spinal cord or by intravenous administration of an agent known to block the action of norepinephrine. Thus the investigators concluded that the central nervous system increases blood pressure by increasing the activity of the sympathetic nervous system.

Buckley and his colleagues have shown that destruction of a portion of the brain called the subnucleus medialis, which is located in the midbrain, abolishes the blood pressure response. Other investigators have shown this area to be involved in the control of peripheral resistance to blood flow.

According to Buckley, angiotensin I also increases the blood pressure when injected into the brain. He does not yet know whether this is a direct effect or whether the angiotensin I is first converted into the octapeptide.

Angiotensin II does not have to be injected directly into the brain in order to produce its effects; however, it is somewhat surprising that a peptide of this size would cross the blood-brain barrier, which prevents the movement of many substances from the circulatory system to the brain or spinal cord. Buckley, in his early experiment with dogs, injected the material into the circulatory system. And Carlos Ferrario of the Cleveland Clinic Foundation observed a significant increase in blood pressure in dogs when he injected the octapeptide into an artery leading directly to the brain.

Experiments in Ferrario's laboratory and those of other investigators indicate that another region of the brain, the area postrema, is also involved in regulating blood pressure. Destruction of this area, which is located in the medulla at the base of the brain, prevents the increased blood pressure in response to angiotensin injection. The area postrema is located in a part of the brain that is devoid of a blood-brain barrier, and angiotensin II should have easy access to it. Moreover, there are connections between the area postrema and the nucleus tractus solitarii, a relay station through which pass the nerve fibers from the baroreceptors.

These receptors, which are present in certain major arteries are activated when blood pressure increases. Impulses from the baroreceptor neurons cause the sympathetic neurons that evoke vasoconstriction to stop or slow their firing and thus produce a decrease in blood pressure. Ferrario says that the area postrema may serve as a gate through which angiotensin reaches neurons in the solitary tract and modifies the signals in such a way that sympathetic neurons with which they connect fail to stop firing. The sympathetic neurons would continue to signal the arterioles to constrict even if this response were inappropriate.

Not everyone agrees that angiotensin can cross the blood-brain barrier, but it may not have to. Investigators, including Jacques Genest of the Clinical Research Institute of Montreal and Detlev Ganten of the University of Heidelberg, Germany, have evidence that suggests that angiotensin is synthesized in the brain. The organ contains angiotensins I and II, renin, and the precursor of the angiotensins. Renin is a protein and cannot pass from the blood to the brain.

Some of the evidence concerning the role of the nucleus tractus solitarii in controlling blood pressure comes from the work of Donald Reis and Nobutaka Doba at Cornell University Medical College. These investigators found that, when this portion of the brain is destroyed, rats develop severe hypertension and die of congestive heart failure within a few hours of the operation. Reis and Doba think that the hypertension is due to selective activation of sympathetic neurons that elicit vasoconstriction. They have shown that the blood vessels of the skin, muscles, and internal organs constrict but that other effects of the sympathetic nervous system are absent in the animals. Destruction of the tract apparently prevents the inhibition of the sympathetic neurons by the baroreceptors, so that the sympathetic neurons continue firing even when the blood pressure is already elevated. But Reis says the effects of the central lesions are more severe than those produced by simple severing of the baroreceptor nerve fibers and thinks that additional inhibitory control mechanisms may be interrupted.

Because rats die so rapidly after destruction of the tract, they are not a good model for chronic hypertension. With Marc Nathan, also of Cornell University Medical College, Reis recently produced the lesions in the brains of cats. The animals survive with moderate, but persistent hypertension. Their blood pressures also fluctuate much more than those of normal animals in response to stimuli that elicit changes in blood pressure. The Cornell investigators produced similar changes in cats by using a chemical to selectively destroy certain neurons (those releasing norepinephrine) that innervate the nucleus tractus solitarii. Reis says that this result indicates that chemical imbalances in the brain can produce chronic hypertension.

One of the reasons for the interest in the relationship between the nervous system and hypertension is the widespread although unproven belief that stress causes chronic hypertension. Stress is known to evoke transient increases in blood pressure. But the question is whether that elevated pressure can become chronic if the stress is maintained over long periods of time. This could be the case if the elevated pressure produces biochemical or structural alterations in the blood vessels.

Some investigators, including Reis and M. Samir Amer of the Mead Johnson Research Center, have observed changes in the concentration of cyclic nucleotides in the aortas of rats with chronic hypertension. Certain neurotransmitters released by neurons of the autonomic nervous system in response to stress and other stimuli are thought to produce their effects by causing increases or decreases in the concentrations of these cyclic nucleotides in the target cells, including smooth muscle cells. The changes observed by the investigators are in the direction that would be expected if the smooth muscle of the vessel walls was becoming more rigid and more resistant to blood flow. If the changes were sustained, the result might be an increase in blood pressure.

Although the renin-angiotensin-aldosterone system may be getting the most attention from investigators of hypertension, these are not the only substances thought to be involved in the regulation of blood pressure. The prostaglandins are also being studied. This family of lipid hormones participates in a number of processes in the body. The situation with regard to their effects on blood pressure regulation is unclear, however, because some prostaglandins act to decrease blood pressure while others increase it.

According to John McGiff of the University of Tennessee Center of the Health Sciences and John Vane of the Wellcome Research Laboratories in Beckenham, England, prostaglandin E_2 (PGE_2) tends to decrease blood pressure by counteracting the angiotensin-induced constriction of the arteries and arterioles. It has been known for some time that responses to angiotensin II diminish when it is administered repeatedly or for prolonged periods of time. McGiff and Vane think that this result occurs because angiotensin stimulates the production of PGE_2.

Infusion of angiotensin II into anesthetized dogs at first decreases the flow of blood through the animals' kidneys, but the flow begins to return to normal even as the infusion is continued. McGiff and Vane showed that the production of PGE_2 by the kidney increases at the same time as does the blood flow. Inhibition of prostaglandin synthesis by the drug indomethacin prevented the increase. Moreover, indomethacin decreased renal blood flow in the absence of added angiotensin, and doses of angiotensin that were without effect before inhibition of prostaglandin synthesis decreased renal blood flow in the presence of the inhibitor.

McGiff and Vane suggest that maintenance of the rate of blood flow through the kidney when an animal is stressed depends partially on the continuous synthesis of PGE_2 and that, in the absence of that synthesis, the activity of substances that constrict blood vessels is potentiated. A similar situation could be occurring in the arteries and arterioles, which also secrete PGE_2 in the response to angiotensin. Thus, a decline in the synthesis of PGE_2 could contribute to the development of hypertension.

The next question that arises is what could cause such a decline. McGiff and his colleagues have evidence that the answer might be a deficiency of kinins (Figure 17). Kinins are small peptides that lower blood pressure by increasing secretion of water and sodium ions by the kidney and by causing the dilation of blood vessels. The best

H-Arg-Pro-Pro-Gly-Phe-Ser-Pro-Phe-Arg-OH   (a)

H-Lys-Arg-Pro-Pro-Gly-Phe-Ser-Pro-Phe-Arg-OH   (b)

Figure 17.   Structures of bradykinin (a) and lysyl-bradykinin (b).

known kinins are bradykinin and lysyl-bradykinin. According to McGiff, bradykinin stimulates PGE_2 release by the kidney and the arteries, and the prostaglandin appears to mediate some effects of the kinin.

The enzyme kallikrein produces the kinins by catalyzing the splitting of a large peptide found in blood. Harry Margolius, now at the Medical College of South Carolina, Ronald Geller of the National Heart, Lung, and Blood Institute and their colleagues have found that patients with hypertension secrete less kallikrein in their urine than do persons with normal blood pressure. A deficiency of the enzyme should result in a lack of kinins. Another pertinent observation in this regard is that mean urinary kallikrein concentrations are lower for black than for white children, according to Margolius and his colleagues, even though the black children had normal blood pressures. The incidence of high blood pressure is much greater in the black population than among whites. Moreover, the investigators found that the mean blood pressures of the families with low mean kallikrein concentrations in urine were significantly higher than those for families with high kallikrein concentrations. These results suggest that a biochemical defect, possibly of genetic origin, may predispose to the development of hypertension.

Whereas PGE_2 appears to decrease blood pressure, the prostaglandin $PGF_{2\alpha}$ increases it. The latter compound does this by constricting the veins and thus enhancing the return of blood to the heart. This in turn increases cardiac output. Consequently, more blood is pumped into the arteries and the arterial pressure increases. $PGF_{2\alpha}$ may also stimulate cardiac output by a direct effect on the heart.

The net effect of the prostaglandins on blood pressure would appear to depend on which one is predominant at a given time. And this could depend on their relative rates of synthesis. McGiff points out that $PGF_{2\alpha}$ may be synthesized from PGE_2 as a result of the activity of the enzymes PGE 9-ketoreductase. He suggests that this enzyme could play a regulatory role, with an increase in its activity favoring an increase in blood pressure and a decrease disposing to a decline in blood pressure.

Whether inhibiting prostaglandin production by administering indomethacin to the intact animal will increase or decrease blood pressure is unclear. Indomethacin is sometimes used as a substitute for aspirin, but McGiff says that there is no evidence that it increases the blood pressure of individuals taking it. McGiff and his colleagues found that the drug did increase the blood pressure of rabbits and dogs.

On the other hand, Jürgen Frölich, John Oates, and their colleagues at Vanderbilt University found that indomethacin decreased blood pressure in a small number of hypertensive patients and in normal individuals. They gave the drug to human volunteers because they and other investigators had evidence that prostaglandins stimulate the release of renin by the kidneys. This would favor angiotensin production and should increase blood pressure. Thus, Frölich and Oates hypothesized that indomethacin should decrease blood pressure in the patients. The discrepancies between their results and those of McGiff obviously require further clarification.

The difficulty in sorting out the role of the prostaglandins in regulating blood pressure exemplifies the problems faced by all the investigators. The whole area of research is clouded by the fact that regulation is achieved by the interaction of several different systems. The researchers agree that disturbances in any one system may cause chronic hypertension, but as yet they have been unable to clarify the contribution of each.

Meanwhile, clinicians who seek to treat hypertension have a more practical problem to worry about — that is, the failure of many patients to stick to the therapeutic regimen prescribed for them. According to a recent estimate from the NHLBI, less than one-third of the hypertensive persons in the United States have their condition under adequate control, despite the availability of an easy, noninvasive technique for detecting high blood pressure and of effective therapies. One reason for patient noncompliance is that hypertension does not usually cause symptoms until the condition has progressed to the point where damage has occurred in the form of atherosclerosis, kidney impairment, heart disease, or stroke. The untreated patient may feel fine and not want to bother with therapy which can be inconvenient, expensive, and have unpleasant side effects.

Therapy for hypertension usually includes treatment with one or more drugs, often in conjunction with a weight-reducing diet for overweight patients. It may also be necessary for patients to restrict their salt intake. Diets are rarely considered enjoyable, and many of the drugs are associated with side effects such as weakness or drowsiness and, in some cases, impotence. These usually diminish with time or can be overcome by adjusting the dosage or substituting one drug for another, but a patient may simply feel better when not taking the drugs and thus drop out of therapy before the optimum drug combination is found. This is one reason why investigators would like to develop more scientific methods for tailoring therapies to fit a given individual's needs. Other factors that may contribute to this problem of patient noncompliance are the complicated schedules that may be required when two or more drugs are prescribed and the fact that the treatment, which must often be continued for life, can cost a lot of money over long periods of time.

The following are among the drugs now used:

• Diuretics to increase the excretion of salt and water and thus deplete the blood volume. Some common diuretics are the sulfonamides, spironolactone, and furosemide.

• Agents that act directly on the blood vessels to produce dilation. These include hydralazine and minoxidil.

• Agents that produce vasodilation by counteracting the vasoconstricting action of the sympathetic nervous system. These include guanethidine, bethanidine, debrisoquine, and reserpine.

• Agents to decrease renin production by the kidney and thus decrease constriction of the blood vessels. Some of the drugs that are thought to decrease renin act in more than one way. This is true for reserpine, for example, and for methyldopa, which also acts through the nervous system. Propranolol may be given in combination with certain of the other drugs in order to counteract their side effects, and may have the additional effect of lowering renin output.

Physicians, who may fail to prescribe the effective drugs that are available now, often share the blame for inadequate control of a patient's hypertension, according to members of the National High Blood Pressure Coordinating Committee. Equally important is the need for the physician to communicate to the patient the necessity of continuing treatment, to follow up on the patient's condition, and to adjust the therapy in response to any problems that may arise.

There are a number of programs sponsored by the government

and private organizations aimed at educating both the public and the medical profession about the importance of all patients receiving adequate treatment for hypertension. One of these is the National High Blood Pressure Education Program. This program, which involves a number of federal and state agencies and private organizations, is coordinated by the NHLBI. Its functions include the collection of information about the current state of hypertension therapy, the dissemination of the information to health professionals, and then working with the professionals to set standards for treatment of the disease.

The American Heart Association, through its local chapters and in conjunction with civic groups, sponsors free clinics to screen for persons who have high blood pressure. Those with hypertension are urged to see their physicians or are directed to appropriate clinics for treatment. When possible, volunteers check back with the persons to determine whether or not they are receiving treatment. High blood pressure is one major health problem that can be solved, but only if the person who has it obtains treatment, and then sticks with it.

IV

Diagnosis and Treatment

12

DIAGNOSIS AND TREATMENT
A New Era

Many people view a diagnosis of heart disease as a death knell. Even medically sophisticated people have hesitated to see a cardiologist when they first experienced symptoms suggestive of heart disease, fearing to hear or refusing to believe that they do indeed have it. Others have delayed seeking medical help even when they were in the throes of a heart attack.

To some extent, this fear of heart disease is well founded. After all, nearly 700,000 people in the United States die of heart attacks each year and two-thirds of heart attack victims die before they reach a hospital. But medical researchers are becoming increasingly optimistic that they can reduce this toll. The first step is to diagnose the disease, and enormous progress has recently been made in the development of noninvasive diagnostic methods. This progress promises to facilitate attempts to decide which treatments are optimal for different groups of heart disease patients. Since the methods are noninvasive, they can be used repeatedly on patients to follow the progress of heart disease and to facilitate research on treatments and preventive methods. New treatments, moreover, are constantly being proposed, and some show promise in extending lives and alleviating symptoms of heart disease patients.

According to Walter Henry of the National Heart, Lung, and Blood Institute, "We are in the midst of a revolution in diagnosing heart disease — a revolution that is not generally appreciated." For example, cardiologists now routinely use ultrasound (echocardiograms) in diagnosis. But as recently as a decade ago, this technique was viewed with skepticism by most medical researchers. Now, says

Henry, echocardiograms are revealing so much detail of heart structures and movements that many cardiologists are still adjusting to this onslaught of information and are still trying to sort out normal variations from pathologies. Thus they are diagnosing such things as mitral valve prolapse in as many as 20 percent of their patients. Henry, however, who has worked exclusively with echocardiography for nearly a decade, estimates that only about 5 percent of heart patients actually have this valve disorder.

Another example of the rapid pace of progress in noninvasively diagnosing heart disease is the spread of a recently developed technique for making movies of beating hearts while patients rest and while they exercise. The method was developed only about $1\frac{1}{2}$ years ago, but already five companies are marketing equipment to make the movies. Jeffrey Borer of the NHLBI, who is a developer of the method, says that the first company came out with movie-making equipment within 6 months after the technique was reported. The equipment is being purchased by community hospitals as well as by research institutions.

In many situations, the movies of beating hearts provide tremendous diagnostic advantages over conventional methods. For example, the movies are much more sensitive than exercise electrocardiograms in detecting when patients have atherosclerosis severe enough to affect their hearts during exercise. Borer and his colleagues studied 57 patients with exercise electrocardiograms and with the movie technique. Of these patients, only 50 percent had positive electrocardiograms which indicated the presence of heart disease. However, in 90 percent, evidence of blocked coronary arteries showed up during the exercise portions of the movies. These diagnoses were confirmed by coronary angiograms (an invasive and more dangerous technique). According to Borer, the conclusion is that the movies, unlike the electrocardiograms, give neither false positive nor false negative results.

The study of how to treat heart disease patients is not quite in a state of revolution, but rapid progress is nonetheless being made. Medical researchers are becoming optimistic that prompt treatment of heart attack victims may limit the damage to their hearts and that some new drugs may control the dangerous arrhythmias that lead to sudden death.

Among the most promising developments is the discovery that there may be a portion of heart tissue that, if treated rapidly, may recover from heart attack damage. Researchers find that certain drugs can minimize heart attack damage in animals. Moreover, the drugs also seemed useful in limited clinical trials with humans. Now, the NHLBI is planning a full-scale clinical trial of two of these drugs—propranolol and hyaluronidase. According to Michael Mock of the NHLBI, the trial will involve five clinical centers and may include as many as 1000 heart attack patients. The trial participants will be given a drug or a placebo within 18 hours after their heart attacks. The trial investigators will assess the effectiveness of the drugs in several ways, including some of the newer methods of detecting heart damage.

Since 75 percent of heart patients are more than 65 years old, research on the detection and treatment of heart disease has spurred a new interest in how the heart changes with age. Studies of the aging heart are especially important since some conditions that may seem pathological in younger people are normal in the aged. For example, researchers had always thought that hypertension caused three characteristic changes in patient's hearts: increase in the size of the aorta, increase in the size of the left atrium, and thickening of the heart walls. Now Henry and his associates have used echocardiography to show that these changes may not always be due to hypertension. They report that all three changes are normal consequences of aging and that only the heart wall thickening is more pronounced in hypertensives when age is taken into account.

Not all of the current research on detection and treatment of heart disease can yet promise to prolong lives and relieve the suffering of patients. This is especially true for the elderly patients who, until recently, have been given short shrift by medical investigators. But the new research results hold out a great deal of promise for eventual adoption of rational and proven methods of detecting and treating heart disease. Perhaps if the dire consequences of heart disease can be reduced, people's fear of it will also diminish.

13

DETECTION OF HEART DISEASE
Promising New Methods

Many medical researchers believe that the only way to prevent deaths from heart disease is to prevent heart disease. Failing that, the next best thing is to devise effective treatments once heart disease occurs. In some cases, surgery may repair congenital damage or damage due to rheumatic fever. For those who have atherosclerotic heart disease, surgery or drugs may limit the extent of the damage by keeping alive areas of heart muscle that would otherwise die. But before methods of treatment can be used or evaluated, certain questions must be answered: Are the patient's symptoms due to heart disease? If so, what are the extent and location of the damage? What are the effects of the damage on the heart's function? Does the therapy actually limit the extent of the damage?

To answer these questions, safe, accurate, and reliable techniques for detecting damage are necessary. Physicians now tend to rely on chest x-rays, electrocardiograms, and contrast angiograms. The chest x-ray indicates how large the heart is and provides a gross way of assessing the heart's function. For example, it can detect pulmonary edema due to congestive heart failure. The electrocardiogram often provides nonspecific information and is a relatively insensitive indicator of heart abnormalities. For example, an electrocardiogram can usually indicate whether a person is having a heart attack, but gives little information as to the size of the damaged area of the heart.

Contrast angiograms are generally performed when surgery or some other therapies are being contemplated for people who have chest pains (angina pectoris) or who have recently recovered from heart attacks. They provide an indication of the extent of the damage and of how the heart functions, but are somewhat painful, dangerous, and expensive. When an angiogram is made, a catheter is inserted into a person's heart, a radiopaque medium is injected, and x-ray pictures and movies are made. The pictures show where arteries are blocked and how extensive the blockage is. The movies show how the heart functions.

In lieu of these standard methods of detecting damage, some promising new methods are being developed. Most, however, are not yet in clinical use. The newer techniques provide more information than chest x-rays and electrocardiograms and are safer and less uncomfortable than angiograms. Some of these methods involve indirect measurements of damage. For example, a radioimmunoassay developed by Robert Roberts and Burton Sobel of Washington University can be used to detect a specific enzyme, creatine phosphokinase (CPK), released into the blood when heart muscle dies. The most promising methods, however, produce pictures of the heart in which damaged heart tissue and its effects on heart function can be seen.

Pictures of the heart are obtained in several ways. The heart can be labeled with radioactive tracers that emit γ-rays and pictures taken with a scintillation camera that detects γ-radiation. Computerized methods can be used to build up a three-dimensional picture of the heart from x-ray or γ-ray pictures, or high-frequency sound can be beamed at the heart and a picture reconstructed from the reflections of the sound. These methods have different advantages and disadvantages, and they complement, rather than replace, each other. Together they are leading to improved diagnoses, to more accurate prognoses, and to better evaluations of treatments.

In the past few years, scintillation camera images have come into increasing use in diagnosing heart attacks. Some patients admitted to hospitals with symptoms of heart attack may have equivocal electrocardiograms, and the absence of serum enzymes, such as CPK, may not preclude heart damage. In these cases, scintillation camera images have proved extremely useful. Since these images also indicate the extent and location of damage, investigators at several medical centers, including Johns Hopkins University and the University of Texas Medical Center at Dallas, now routinely make images of patients' hearts to diagnose suspected heart disease.

Three ways to detect damage with a scintillation camera have been developed. The first results in a picture of areas of heart muscle that have recently died or been damaged. A radionuclide tracer, such as technetium-99m, is attached to a substance, such as pyrophosphate, that has an affinity for recently damaged heart muscle. Patients are injected intravenously with these tracers. The radionuclide lodges in and emits γ-rays from damaged areas, which then show up as bright areas in the scintillation camera image.

This method has several drawbacks. One difficulty is that small areas of damage, especially those that do not affect the full thickness of a wall of the heart, are not always detected. In recent years it has become clear that clinically important problems can occur when only part of the heart wall is damaged.

Another problem is that conditions other than acute damage to heart tissue can cause the tracers to accumulate. Several groups of researchers find that people with unstable angina pectoris – that is, angina pectoris in which the temporal pattern of pain changes – sometimes accumulate these tracers in their hearts. These people, however, may have no other signs of damage detectable by electrocardiograms or changes in concentrations of serum CPK. B. Leonard Holman and his colleagues at Harvard Medical School report that these tracers apparently bind to tissues that are deprived of oxygen whether or not those tissues are irreversibly damaged. This complicates the problem of separating patients with acute damage, who need intensive care, from those with less severe problems. Important therapeutic decisions may depend on this distinction.

An alternate way to see damaged heart muscle is to look at its complement – healthy heart muscle. In this case, a radioactive tracer consisting of a monovalent cation, such as potassium-43 or thallium-201, is injected intravenously into the patient. These tracers lodge in the heart in proportion to blood flow. Thus, portions of the heart that are deprived of blood as a result of blockage of the coronary arteries show up as blank areas in the scintillation camera image. These blank areas may indicate either recently damaged tissue or tissue damaged by a previous heart attack. Once again, damaged areas that do not affect the entire heart wall may be missed. Recent damage can be distinguished from old when pictures taken with these monovalent cations are compared to pictures taken with radionuclides that concentrate only in recently damaged areas.

The third type of scintillation camera image provides information on how well the heart functions. To provide a radioactive label, a blood pool tracer is injected into the patient. Such a tracer consists of a radionuclide attached to red blood cells or to a substance, such as albumin, that is carried along with the blood and does not lodge in heart tissue. The patient's cardiac cycle is recorded with an electrocardiograph, which, at specific points in the cycle, triggers the scintillation camera to record an image of the heart.

The resulting images of the heart at several points in the cardiac cycle provide information on whether the heart's left ventricle functions properly as a whole and whether all regions of the heart's walls move normally. The left ventricle is of greatest interest because it is the chamber that supplies blood to the major organs of the body and the one that is most commonly damaged by heart disease. Damage to heart muscle, including damage that does not involve the entire heart wall, often causes abnormal wall movements. Thus, determinations of wall movements can indicate dead or severely damaged areas of heart muscle that could not be detected with the other scintillation camera images.

Jeffrey Borer, with Stephen Bacharach and Michael Green at the National Heart, Lung, and Blood Institute and the division of computer technology of the National Institutes of Health, and, independently, Bertram Pitt and William Strauss of Johns Hopkins University Medical School have recently refined this method of imaging the heart. These researchers now make movies of beating hearts rather than still shots. The movies are made with computers that store images taken at closely spaced intervals during the cardiac cycle. The Hopkins and NHLBI groups also use their computers to calculate and display graphically the volume of blood ejected from the heart when it contracts. This is possible because the blood is radioactively labeled and so the radioactivity of the heart at any time is a measure of the relative volume of blood in the heart. The ejection fraction — that is, the percentage of blood ejected in a single beat — is an indicator of left ventricular function (Figure 18).

In addition to using scintillation camera images to diagnose heart attacks, investigators are using these images to detect heart damage in people without symptoms who have normal resting cardiac functions and in people with angina pectoris. Borer and his colleagues are among those using their movies for this purpose. These researchers first make a movie of a person's heart and calculate the heart's ejection fraction while the person is at rest. Then they

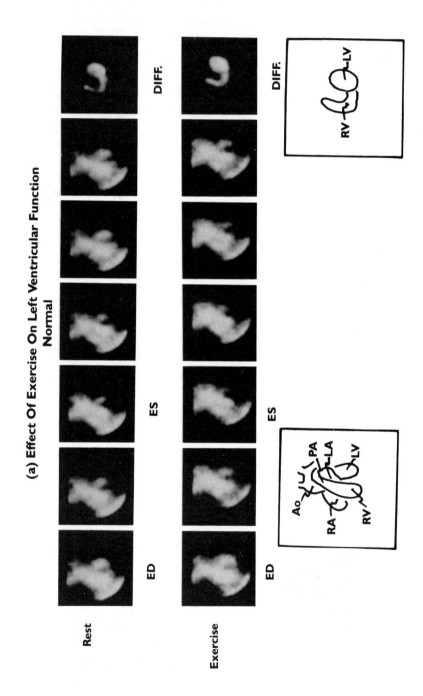

(a) Effect Of Exercise On Left Ventricular Function

Normal

(b) Effect Of Exercise On Left Ventricular Function
Coronary Artery Disease

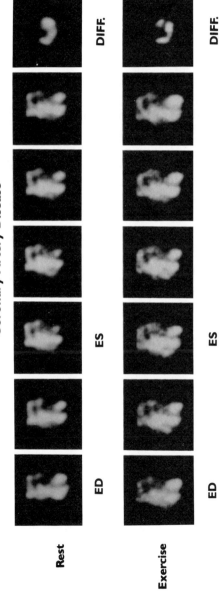

Figure 18. Effect of exercise on left ventricular function. (a) Selected frames, in sequence, of a movie made with a scintillation camera of a normal subject's heart at rest (upper) and during maximal exercise (lower); *ED* denotes end-diastolic frame; *ES*, end-systolic frame; *DIFF*, difference image (created by electronic substitution of end-systolic counts from end-dyastolic counts); *Ao*, aorta; *PA*, pulmonary artery; *RA*, right atrium; *RV*, right ventricle; *LA*, left atrium; and *LV*, left ventricle. (b) Selected frames, in sequence, of a movie made of a patient with three occluded coronary arteries at rest (upper) and during maximal exercise (lower). [Source: J. S. Borer, S. L. Bacharach, and M. V. Green, National Heart, Lung, and Blood Institute, reprinted with the permission of the *New England Journal of Medicine*]

repeat the process while the person is exercising. When they compare the two movies, they can see previously undetected regions of left ventricular dysfunctions that occur only during exercise. As Borer points out, this evaluation provides information that cannot be obtained from other methods, such as exercise electrocardiograms. He and others find that such electrocardiograms result in large proportions of both false positive and false negative diagnoses of coronary heart disease.

People with angina pectoris have coronary arteries that are so narrowed that, although they may carry enough blood to the heart when the person is at rest, they cannot supply the increased blood flow that is needed during exercise. When these people exercise, areas of their hearts are deprived of oxygen and they develop chest pain.

Pitt, Strauss, and Ian Bailey of Johns Hopkins University Medical School find that, because thallium-201 labels only areas of the heart that are well supplied with blood, it can be used to diagnose people with angina pectoris. Patients whose hearts are labeled with this tracer exercise, then rest, during which time scans are made. Heart muscle that is deprived of blood during exercise then becomes evident.

Another use of scintillation camera images is to evaluate treatments of heart disease patients. Borer is using his movies of beating hearts to see whether people who have coronary bypass operations subsequently have improved left ventricular functions and whether nitroglycerin improves heart function during exercise. Pitt and Strauss are using their movies to see whether nitroglycerin improves heart function at rest.

Scintillation camera images are also being used to obtain information that is useful for making prognoses. Robert Chisholm of Harvard Medical School and Holman evaluated 100 patients with suspected acute infarctions. They labeled the recently damaged muscle with a radionuclide. By determining how much of a patient's heart took up this tracer, Holman and Chisholm were able to distinguish low-risk from high-risk patients. These investigators claim that this ability should enable them to reduce the hospitalization times of low-risk patients and to identify the high-risk patients who would benefit from more intensive treatment.

Although the scintillation camera images of the heart have numerous advantages over electrocardiograms and angiograms, they also have drawbacks that limit their uses. For example, the radioactive tracers have half-lives on the order of hours. This makes it impossible to make serial images that show the location of the damage during the first few hours after a heart attack begins (when most damage occurs). Serial images would be most useful at that time since they would provide a means to monitor the progress of the damage. (Although the movies do constitute serial images, they indicate heart function but not the location of damage.) Another problem is that these images constitute two-dimensional projections of the three-dimensional heart. Thus, heart structures are superimposed, making the scintillation camera images difficult to interpret.

Some of these difficulties with scintillation camera images are avoided when images are reconstructed by computerized tomography. This technique is still a research tool for imaging the heart, but indications are that it will soon come into clinical use.

Computerized tomography is based on a mathematical method for constructing a three-dimensional image from two-dimensional projections. The projections are taken from several angles, and then the information is processed by a computer to produce three-dimensional pictures in the form of a series of two-dimensional cross sections.

This method of computerized reconstruction has come into widespread use for making pictures of stationary organs, such as the brain. But it has had to be modified before it could be applied to a moving organ such as the heart. Difficulties with imaging the heart occur because, as the machine moves from position to position to take pictures from different angles, both the shape and position of the heart change. This movement results in a blurred picture.

The beating heart is not a problem in one type of computerized tomography that results in such low-resolution pictures that heart movements are not noticed. The method, however, uses tracers with properties that compensate for this low resolution. This technique is being used successfully by Michael Ter-Pogossian, Edward Weiss, Sobel, and their associates at Washington University, and independently, by Gordon Brownell and his associates at Massachusetts General Hospital.

These investigators label the heart with positron-emitting isotopes and then use a machine that scans the heart and detects γ-rays emitted when these positrons collide with electrons. Because of the low intensity of the emitted γ-rays, the resulting images have a

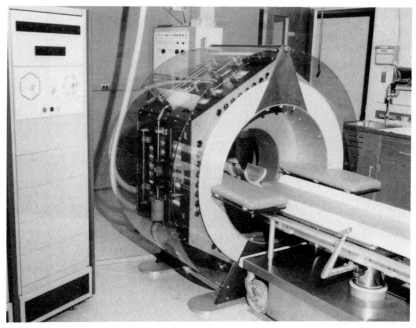

Figure 19. A positron-emission tomographic system. This machine can provide simultaneously images of seven slices of the body or the head and has been used to obtain images of the heart. [Source: Michael M. Ter-Pogossian, Washington University School of Medicine]

resolution of only 1 centimeter, as compared to 1 millimeter with conventional computerized x-ray techniques. Ter-Pogossian, Brownell, and their associates have, however, chosen positron-emitting isotopes with several advantages which make up for this lack of resolution (Figure 19).

The positron-emitting isotopes used are isotopes of carbon and nitrogen. These isotopes can be incorporated into compounds such as palmitate or ammonia, which are taken up more readily by healthy than by oxygen-deprived tissues. For example, ^{11}C-palmitate, which is used by the Washington University group, is taken up and metabolized almost exclusively by the heart.

Another advantage of the positron-emitting isotopes is that they have very short half-lives — about 10 minutes for ^{13}N and 20 minutes for ^{11}C. This means that serial images of the heart can be obtained and the progress of damage during the course of a few hours followed. The short half-lives, however, mean that the isotopes must be used almost as soon as they are produced. Since they are produced in cyclotrons, the cost currently limits the number of medical centers where they are available.

More conventional computerized tomography relies on the transmission of x-rays through body tissues to produce the two-dimensional cross-sectional images of body organs. Structures and damaged areas of the heart can be seen because they differ in the degree to which they attenuate x-rays. (Patients are usually injected with a contrast medium before their hearts are imaged, however, so as to enhance these attenuation differences.) The x-rays are about 1000 times more intense than the positron-emitting isotopes, thus resulting in higher resolution images than emission tomography.

To get around the problem of the heart's movements and still produce clear pictures with transmission tomography, investigators are following two different strategies. The first is to monitor the cardiac cycle and to make images only at certain points of the cycle. This is a difficult technique, however, which is still being developed (Figure 20).

The second strategy is to position numerous x-ray sources around the chest and then to produce the two-dimensional images from all the requisite angles simultaneously. A prototype of a machine that would do this was built by Earl Wood and his associates at the Mayo Clinic. They are currently using the machine on dogs, but plan to use it soon on people. With this machine, they can produce 60 three-dimensional images of a dog's heart per second and display the images as a movie of various cross sections of a beating heart. They will use this technique to measure blood flow through the coronary arteries of patients and to see, with a 1-millimeter resolution, which areas of patients' hearts are supplied with and which are deprived of blood.

Despite its advantages for viewing heart structures and movements, computerized tomography is an expensive technique. In some cases, similar information may be obtained at much less expense with ultrasound imaging.

Ultrasound – that is, sound with frequencies greater than 20,000 hertz – has come into extensive clinical use within the past few years. Heart structures and movements can be detected when pulses of ultrasound are beamed at the heart. Most of this sound passes through body tissues, but some is reflected back each time the beam hits the interface between soft tissues of different compositions. By

I

II

III

IV

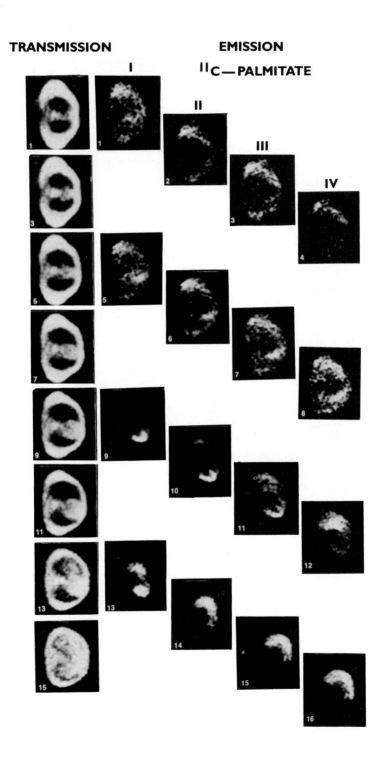

recording the time required for a beam to enter the body and be reflected back from a particular structure, medical scientists can estimate the distance of that structure from the source of the sound and chart how the structure moves with time. In that way, they can diagnose such things as congenital heart defects, enlargement of the heart due to congestive heart failure or hypertension, and defects in heart valves.

Almost all current ultrasound techniques in cardiology result in one-dimensional images. The beam is moved from place to place and provides information on the manner in which different points on the heart move. The graphs of these movements are useful in assessing the overall structure and function of the heart but most often do not show segmental damage, such as that resulting from coronary artery disease.

Several groups of investigators have developed means of obtaining two-dimensional images of the heart with ultrasound. A problem in going from one to two dimensions arises from the heart's movements, which make it difficult to move a transducer across a person's chest, store the information as it is obtained, and finally display the information in two dimensions. Instead, it is necessary to sweep a beam across the heart more rapidly than the heart beats. Walter Henry and his associates at the NHLBI and Harvey Feigenbaum and his associates at the University of Indiana do this with a transducer that mechanically sweeps through an arc of 30° to 45° at a rate of 30 times per second. An alternate method is to use an array of transducers to electronically produce a wedge of sound. This is the method of Joseph Kisslo and his associates at Duke University and of James Meindl of Stanford University.

The two-dimensional images look like slices of the heart. Investigators can see valves open and close and can produce slices perpendicular to the long axis of the heart. These images are especially useful in the diagnosis of congenital heart defects in which the structures of the heart are displaced from their normal positions. Kisslo and his associates are also using their two-dimensional pic-

---

Figure 20. Photographs of a normal beating human heart. The "transmission" images were obtained by transmission tomography. The "emission" images were obtained by positron-emission tomography. The patient's heart was labeled with ^{11}C-palmitate. [Source: Michael M. Ter-Pogossian, Washington University School of Medicine]

tures to detect abnormal movements of the left ventricular walls produced by areas of dead or damaged heart muscle.

Since ultrasound can be used to produce two-dimensional images of the heart from a number of different angles, it is possible to gather enough information to construct a three-dimensional image of the heart. Although they are not yet able to display three-dimensional images, Meindl and his associates can collect two-dimensional images from all the angles necessary to construct them. At present, they use a computer to calculate heart volumes during the cardiac cycle from this information. Heart volumes in turn provide estimates of the volume of blood ejected when the heart contracts, which indicates left ventricular function.

Ultrasound, as used diagnostically, does not seem to harm subjects, and its technology is progressing rapidly. This technique cannot be used on everyone, however. Good images can be made of children's hearts, but images of adult hearts vary in quality. As much as 15 to 20 percent of the adult population have physiological traits, such as unusual chest wall configurations, that preclude the use of ultrasound.

All of the newer methods of viewing the heart represent attempts to detect damage, but the methods differ as to what effects of damage they detect. The monovalent cation tracers detect biochemical changes that occur when heart muscle is damaged. Radionuclide tracers such as thallium-201 detect defects in blood flow to damaged areas. Positron emission tomography that utilizes labeled palmitate detects changes in the metabolism of damaged tissue. Transmission tomography detects changes in the attenuation of x-rays by damaged myocardium. And ultrasound measures the movements and the dimensions of the heart. It is not yet clear which combination of these variables is most useful for the assessment of damage. However, these newer techniques together yield more information less dangerously than any combination of techniques used in the past.

14

AFTER THE HEART ATTACK
Limiting the Damage

Although researchers have identified at least some of the steps that would have to be taken to reduce the heart attack toll, it is still far too high. Of the more than 640,000 heart attack deaths per year in the United States, 70 percent occur outside the hospital. For those victims who manage to reach the hospital, however, chances of survival have been improved by coronary care units and the availability of drugs to control the potentially fatal disturbances in heart rhythms that may result from damage to cardiac muscle. Cardiologists anticipate that survival rates will be further improved by therapies that limit the amount of cardiac muscle killed as a result of blockage of the coronary arteries.

This optimism contrasts with the pessimism of previous years. Until the 1960s, it was thought that when the blood supply to a portion of the heart muscle was sharply reduced, the muscle died and there was little or nothing that anyone could do about it. However, more recent research has shown that, although this might be true for part of the area affected, there is a borderline zone that may recover. Moreover, the evidence indicates that the extent of the recovery can be influenced by the treatment the patient receives. It is not only necessary to avoid harmful therapies but it appears possible to institute beneficial ones.

The basis for much of the current research is the understanding that blockage of one or more of the three major coronary arteries by atherosclerotic lesions or blood clots rarely cuts off all blood flow to the affected portion of the heart. Collateral arteries, which are small vessels branching from nearby open arteries, can carry some blood to the tissue, but the flow is reduced so that the supply of oxygen is less than the demand for it. Tissue that is not receiving an adequate blood supply is called "ischemic." If the imbalance between oxygen supply and demand is high or persists for a long enough time, the ischemic tissue may die. The dead area is called an "infarct." The experiments of Robert Jennings, Keith Reimer, and James Lowe of Duke University Medical School have shown that severely ischemic tissue dies very rapidly but that the affected area also contains moderately ischemic tissue that may recover. Consequently, many of the strategies to limit infarct size aim to increase the supply of oxygen to the heart, to decrease the demand for it, or, if possible, to do both.

One of the pioneers in this research is Eugene Braunwald, working first at the University of California at San Diego (UCSD) and more recently at Harvard Medical School. According to Braunwald, John Ross of UCSD, and Peter Maroko, who is now at Harvard, the most important factors that influence the heart's demand for oxygen are tension development (degree of stretch in the heart wall), the contractility of cardiac muscle (how fast and forcefully the muscle fibers can shorten), and the heart rate; increases in all of these increase oxygen consumption.

In experiments on dogs, the investigators found that drugs, some of which are used to treat heart attack victims, may in some circumstances actually cause infarct enlargement. This is true for isoproterenol, for example. Isoproterenol increases the amount of blood pumped by the heart by increasing contractility and the heart rate. Although increasing the cardiac output might appear to be desirable for a patient whose heart is pumping poorly after a heart attack, the results of the Braunwald group indicate that there is also danger of causing the size of the infarct to increase.

The encouraging result from a number of laboratories, including Braunwald's, is that certain therapies can prevent extension of the area of dead tissue. A smaller infarct means that the risk of dangerous arrhythmias and death are decreased, and the patient's chances of leading a more normal life with less disability are increased.

Most of the research thus far has been carried out on animals, but a few drugs, including nitroglycerin, hyaluronidase, and propranolol, have undergone preliminary trials in humans. The investigators think that the early experiments have been successful enough to warrant more extensive clinical trials.

Experiments by Stephen Epstein, Jeffrey Borer, and their colleagues at the National Heart, Lung, and Blood Institute showed that administration of nitroglycerin (Figure 21) to dogs decreased the size of infarcts produced by tying off one of the coronary arteries. The drug also lowered the susceptibility of the hearts to ventricular fibrillation, a dangerous heart arrhythmia.

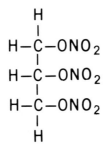

Figure 21. Structure of nitroglycerin.

The NHLBI investigators and another team of cardiologists at Johns Hopkins University Medical School have recently tested the effects of nitroglycerin on a limited number of heart attack patients. Both groups found that the drug improved heart function and reduced the extent of the injury caused by ischemia. The researchers used electrocardiograms (ECG's) to assess the extent of the damage. The magnitude of the deviation from normal of a certain ECG abnormality is known to correlate with the size of the ischemic area, and Braunwald and Maroko have shown that it also correlates with eventual infarct size. Reduction in the magnitude of the abnormality as observed by the investigators following nitroglycerin treatment suggests that the drug has acted to reduce the extent of the damage.

The results of the two groups were similar in that both showed that nitroglycerin alone improved the condition of patients with failing hearts. (Not all heart attack victims suffer heart failure.) However, the NHLBI investigators found that the effects of nitroglycerin were unpredictable in patients without heart failure unless they were also given a drug to counteract the drop in blood pressure and the rise in heart rate it elicited. Although the drug potentiated the effects of nitroglycerin in these patients, it diminished the effects of nitroglycerin in patients with heart failure. On the other hand, Bertram Pitt of Johns Hopkins University Medical School said that their study indicated that a drug to raise blood pressure reversed the beneficial effects of nitroglycerin in both groups of patients.

The reason for the difference is not clear, although the two teams of investigators administered the nitroglycerin by different routes. The NHLBI investigators gave the patients nitroglycerin tablets to be held under the tongue, whereas the Johns Hopkins workers injected the drug intravenously. Pitt says that with the latter route it is easier to control the dosage to avoid large drops in blood pressure or increases in heart rate. Nevertheless, Epstein says that these effects make it necessary to exercise extreme caution in the administration of nitrogylcerin to patients without heart failure no matter what route of administration is used.

For many years clinicians feared that attempts to treat any acute heart attack patient with nitroglycerin would do more harm than good, even though the drug was an established and successful treatment for angina pectoris, a condition in which an individual experiences chest pain during exertion because the coronary arteries have become too narrow to supply adequate blood to the heart in times of increased oxygen demand. Because nitroglycerin increases the heart rate, it could increase oxygen consumption by cardiac muscle. And lowering the blood pressure could decrease the flow of blood through the coronary arteries, if not all of them are blocked. These effects are just the opposite of those desired.

Moreover, the hypotensive action of nitroglycerin might put the patient in greater jeopardy from "pump failure," which occurs if the damaged heart cannot pump effectively enough to maintain blood pressure. As the blood pressure drops the heart muscle receives still less blood, pumps even less efficiently, and the vicious cycle may result in death.

Prediction of the effects of blood pressure alterations can be complicated because a decrease would also lower the work done by the heart and thus its demand for oxygen. For example, in an early experiment, Burton Sobel and his colleagues at the Washington University School of Medicine showed that using the drug trimethaphan to lower the blood pressure of heart attack victims who have hypertension reduced their short-term mortality rate and the size of their infarcts in comparison to those of controls. Since a particular therapy may produce opposing effects on the cardiovascular system, the net effect often depends on the patient's condition. Careful evaluation is needed to determine whether the balance between the effects will be beneficial or harmful.

Although nitroglycerin appears to be a therapy with a beneficial balance, the mechanism by which it limits infarct size is uncertain. Epstein and his associates have evidence that the drug increases the flow of blood through the collateral arteries to the ischemic area. He also thinks, as does the Johns Hopkins group, that nitroglycerin decreases the work of the heart.

Investigators have known for sometime that the drug decreases the amount of blood returned to the heart by dilating the veins so that the vessels contain more blood. This would decrease the pressure inside the left ventricle (the large chamber of the heart that pumps blood to all parts of the body except the lungs, which receive their blood from the right ventricle). The Johns Hopkins investigators have observed such a decrease after nitroglycerin treatment. The lower pressure would reduce the tension on the ventricular walls and the oxygen demand of the heart.

Braunwald and Maroko are encouraged by the results of their clinical trials with the enzyme hyaluronidase. Although the number of treated and control patients was small — a total of approximately 100 in two studies — Braunwald says that analysis of the ECG's of the control patients and those treated with the enzyme indicates that the agent is effective in reducing the amount of heart muscle that is destroyed after a heart attack. (The researchers had previously shown that it would have the effect in dogs with occluded coronary arteries.)

The mode of action of hyaluronidase is still uncertain. The enzyme breaks down hyaluronic acid, which serves as the cement that holds connective tissue together. Braunwald hypothesizes that this may facilitate the diffusion of nutrients through the extracellular space to cells in the area of reduced blood flow. Experiments with dogs showed that the amount of hyaluronic acid between cells in the ischemic area decreases after the animals are treated with the enzyme. Other animal experiments indicated that the enzyme diminishes the damage to the small blood vessels of the heart after a coronary occlusion. Both these effects could help to maintain the oxygen supply to cardiac muscle.

According to Braunwald, the use of hyaluronidase has several advantages. The toxicity of the enzyme is slight, and it only rarely

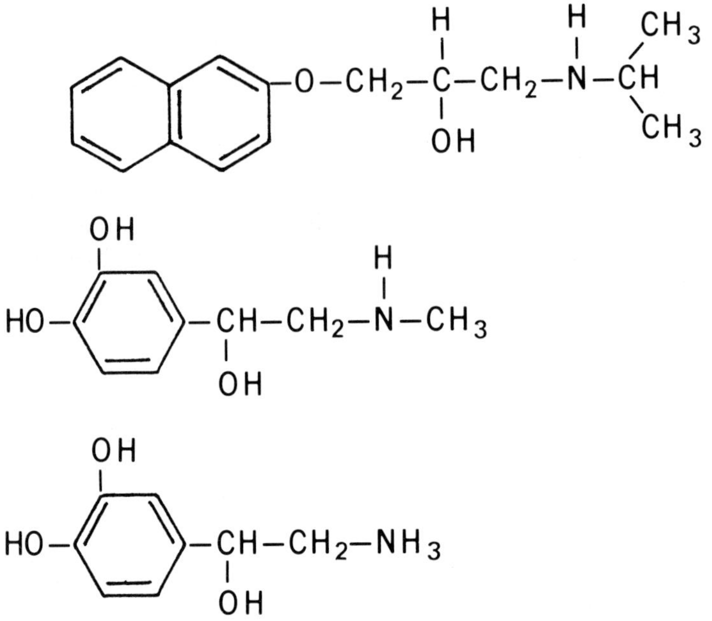

Figure 22. Structures of propranolol (a), epinephrine (b), and norepinephrine (c).

elicits an allergic response. In contrast to nitroglycerin and other drugs being tested for limiting infarct size, hyaluronidase does not have potentially hazardous effects on heart activity or blood pressure. And its use does not require special equipment and patient monitoring that might only be available in major clinical centers.

Propranolol (Figure 22) is a third drug currently being tested in humans for its effects on infarct size. Several investigators, including those in the groups of Braunwald and Jennings, observed that this drug decreased infarct size in dogs. Early results from a number of laboratories indicate that propranolol may do the same in humans.

The drug has several effects that could contribute to this action. It blocks the activity of neurotransmitters, such as epinephrine, that increase heart rate and cardiac contractility and stimulate a variety of biochemical reactions; propranolol thus decreases oxygen consumption by the heart, but it is not clear whether its effects on cell death are due to decreased oxygen consumption or to blockage of the direct effects of the neurotransmitters on certain reactions in the ischemic cells. The evidence concerning whether or not the drug also increases blood flow to ischemic heart muscle is equivocal. Pitt and his co-workers found that it did, whereas Jennings found that it did not.

Drugs are not the only means of influencing the heart's oxygen consumption and supply. Mechanical counterpulsation techniques are being explored in several laboratories. In one such technique, called intra-aortic balloon counterpulsation, a balloon is inserted into the aorta, the main artery leading out of the heart. The balloon is inflated when the heart is at rest between contractions. This is the time when blood flow through the coronary arteries is strongest. Inflating the balloon raises the pressure in the arteries and, as a result increases the heart's blood supply. The balloon is deflated just before contraction begins in order to decrease the pressure against which the heart contracts and thus makes it easier for the heart to pump blood. Similar results can be achieved with external devices that gently compress the leg muscles and major blood vessels between heart beats and release the compression during contraction.

Investigators still need to learn a lot about the application of strategies to limit infarct size. The question of timing—how soon after a heart attack must a treatment be started and how long must it be continued in order to be effective—is an important one which has not yet been answered, although most cardiologists think that a treatment has a greater chance of success if begun early.

According to Jennings, the time that elapses before irreversible damage occurs is inversely related to the degree of ischemia suffered by the tissue. He has found that the reduction of blood flow produced by tying off one of the coronary arteries of the dog hearts is not uniform throughout the affected area. Part of the area is severely ischemic, which Jennings defines as having blood flow reduced by 85 percent. This portion undergoes irreversible damage in 20 to 60 minutes, and the chances of saving it are slim. On the other hand, mildly ischemic areas (50 to 60 percent reduction of blood flow) are unlikely to suffer any irreversible injury. This leaves the moderately ischemic region (70 to 85 percent reduction of blood flow) as the target of salvage attempts. The onset of irreversible damage in this region, which in the dog constitutes about 30 percent of the ischemic tissue, occurs between 1 and 3 hours after the reduction in flow. Although few of the investigators were able to initiate therapy to minimize infarct size this quickly, they still obtained encouraging results. This is fortunate for heart attack victims, many of whom delay for several hours after the onset of symptoms before seeking help.

When cells are receiving a supply of blood inadequate for their needs, they undergo a variety of biochemical and structural changes. One of the major goals of investigators is the identification of the one or ones that actually cause cell death. They think that this knowledge may help them to design better therapeutic strategies for limiting the damage.

One change that occurs very early is a shift from aerobic (oxygen-requiring) to anaerobic (not requiring oxygen) processes for production of the cell's energy. Another early change is a drop in the pH of the ischemic cells. This occurs partly because lactic acid is the final product of the anaerobic breakdown of glucose, a major energy source for cells, and partly because the cells cannot get rid of their waste products, including the lactic acid and carbon dioxide, when the blood flow has been sharply reduced. Several investigators have shown that the pH drop is more severe when blood flow to the heart is stopped than when the heart is perfused with an oxygen-free fluid. The latter can at least carry off waste products.

Anaerobic processes are much less efficient than those requiring oxygen; they produce only enough energy to keep the cells alive, but not enough to support the contraction of the heart muscle cells. If a large proportion of the muscle cannot contract, the heart may go into failure. However, John Williamson of the University of Pennsylvania Medical School thinks that the drop in intracellular pH causes a decrease in heart contraction even before the chemical energy supplied by the aerobic processes is used up. He and his colleagues have found that both the contractile activity of the heart and the intracellular pH drop very rapidly following restriction of blood flow through the coronary arteries of rats. The concentration of adenosine triphosphate (ATP), the chemical form in which energy for contraction is supplied, falls only slightly during this same period of time and cannot account for the decline in contractility of the muscle.

Arnold Katz, who is now at the Mt. Sinai Medical Center in New York, proposed that a low pH prevents binding of calcium ions by part of the contractile mechanism of muscle cells. Since the calcium binding is a prerequisite for contraction, Williamson thinks that this effect could account for a large part of the decline in the contractility of cardiac muscle that has been deprived of blood.

Williamson and his colleagues have observed that after the reduction of blood flow to heart muscle, the ischemic tissue is composed of islands of cells that are receiving essentially no oxygen surrounded by cells that are getting enough to carry on aerobic reactions. It is possible to distinguish between the two because in the anaerobic state certain compounds that are intimately involved in cellular metabolism become reduced whereas in the aerobic state they are oxidized. The two forms emit fluorescent light of different wavelengths.

Williamson says that the drop in pH causes an intense constriction of the small arteries in the tissue. When flow into some of the small vessels is cut off, there may be increased flow into others. Oxygen cannot diffuse very far in the tissue because cells take it up very avidly. The result will be a patchy distribution of the gas, so that a completely aerobic cell may have a completely anaerobic cell for a neighbor.

According to James Neely of the Milton S. Hershey Medical Center of Pennsylvania State University, the decreased pH and, especially, the buildup of lactic acid also inhibit glycolysis, the anaerobic pathway of glucose oxidation that must supply most of the cell's energy after the oxygen supply is cut off. This would tend to make a bad situation worse. It may be possible to limit infarct size by stimulating glycolysis in cardiac muscle while at the same time inhibiting those metabolic processes that require oxygen.

Alterations in the supply of nutrients to the heart muscle may be the basis for the reduction in infarct size that is sometimes seen in heart attack patients who have been infused with a solution containing glucose, insulin, and potassium ions. D. Sodi-Pollares and his colleagues at the National Heart Institute in Mexico City introduced this therapy in the early 1960s. Since then clinical trials of the regimen have produced mixed results at best. Recently, however, Charles Rackley and his colleagues at the University of Alabama Medical Center reported that infusion with the solution reduced the mortality of heart attack patients during hospitalization. The investigators used three standard diagnostic procedures to assess the severity of the infarcts of the 70 treated and the 64 control patients. Although the severity of infarcts in the two groups was similar, the mortality in the patients treated with the solution was significantly lower than that of the controls. The mortality of the former group was from 35 to 50 percent lower than that predicted on the basis of the severity of their condition.

Rackley thinks that the solution works by reducing the availability of free fatty acids to the heart. The free fatty acids are normally a major source of energy of the heart, but other investigators have shown that the fatty acids, which are present in elevated concentrations after a heart attack, increase the risk of dangerous arrhythmias, increase oxygen consumption by the heart, and depress its ability to contract. The Alabama investigators have shown that the fatty acid concentrations are reduced in the blood of treated patients.

The therapy should also increase the availability of glucose to the heart and its breakdown by glycolysis. However, Neely found that perfusion of ischemic swine hearts with a solution containing glucose and insulin did not increase either their glycolysis or their energy production, although it did increase glucose consumption and glycolysis in normal hearts. In the experiments, the concentrations of fatty acids were kept constant in the perfusion fluids.

Cells from ischemic tissue exhibit several kinds of structural abnormalities, especially in their outer membranes and in subcellular structures such as the mitochondria and lysosomes. Jennings thinks that loss of the ability to regulate cell volume as a result of injury to the outer membrane is an early effect of ischemia that may be the primary cause of irreversible damage. He observed that samples of heart tissue that had been irreversibly damaged by 60 minutes of ischemia swelled markedly when incubated in vitro at both 0° and 37°C; the outer membranes of the cells had holes in them. Neither of these changes occurred in control tissues. In vivo, irreversibly damaged cells swell explosively when their blood supply is reestablished, and these cells also have membrane defects similar to those of the incubated cells.

Jennings thinks that the mitochondrial changes that he and other investigators have observed may be a consequence of the defects in the cellular membrane. For example, the mitochondria of irreversibly damaged heart cells accumulate massive quantities of calcium ions; increased movement of the ions through the defective membrane could contribute to the accumulation. In any event, mitochondrial injury could seriously handicap a cell because these structures produce most of the cell's energy.

When the lysosomes incur damage, as they do during ischemia, they release a variety of enzymes that break down cell components, cause inflammation, and further contribute to cellular injury in the affected region of the heart. Investigators have shown that corticosteroids (steroid hormones that suppress inflammation) can stabilize lysosomal and cellular membranes. Braunwald and Maroko found that the hormones have a beneficial effect on infarct size in dogs. However, the results of trials on humans have been inconsistent.

Sobel and his colleagues found that one of these steroids (methylprednisolone) actually increased infarct size and the frequency of dangerous arrhythmias. On the other hand, John Morrison of the North Shore University Hospital in Manhassett, New York, observed that the steroid decreased infarct size in some patients. The reason for this inconsistency is uncertain. Both investigators waited approximately the same time before beginning therapy, and both used a technique devised by the Sobel group to assay for infarct size.

Measuring infarct size in humans continues to be a problem for the investigators engaged in this work. In animal experiments they can directly measure the infarcts in the control and treated animals. When working with humans, the investigators must use noninvasive techniques that will enable them to determine infarct size. In addition, they must show that the infarct is smaller with therapy than it would have been without. Several noninvasive techniques now being developed do not yet have the resolution or sensitivity to do this job. Consequently, most groups have used the special electrocardiographic methods developed by Braunwald and Maroko or the enzymatic one devised by Sobel and his colleagues.

The latter method depends on the fact that irreversibly damaged heart cells release an enzyme called creatine phosphokinase (CPK) into the bloodstream. According to Sobel, an increase in the concentration of the enzyme in blood indicates that a heart attack has occurred and the size of the increase is correlated with the size of the infarct.

The first techniques for measuring CPK activity suffered from a lack of both sensitivity and specificity. Skeletal muscle and other tissues contain structural variants of CPK which catalyze the same reaction as the cardiac enzyme. These variants may be found in blood. The Washington University group has recently developed a radioimmunoassay specific for the heart variant; the new assay is far more sensitive than the previous method, which measured total enzyme activity. (The brain enzyme variant shares a common structure with the one from heart, but the brain enzyme does not escape into the bloodstream.) Sobel thinks that the sensitivity of the radioimmunoassay may permit diagnosis of heart attacks earlier than was possible with the older method. And early diagnosis is essential if infarct size is to be limited and the probability of recovery from heart attacks is to be increased.

15

SUDDEN DEATH
Strategies for Prevention

Of the 60 percent of heart attack victims who die before reaching a hospital, many succumb to ventricular fibrillation; that is, the large chambers of the heart contract in such a chaotic and uncoordinated manner that the heart stops pumping and cardiac arrest ensues. One of the major lessons emerging from the operations of specialized coronary care units is that prompt treatment of cardiac arrest can restore the heartbeat and pull the patient back from the brink of death. Moreover, many of those resuscitated can live at least as normally as persons who have had heart attacks without ventricular fibrillation.

Ventricular fibrillation is caused by disturbances in the electrical impulses that normally regulate the heart's beating. The likelihood that the disturbances will occur increases with the size of the infarct (dead tissue) that results when blood flow to a portion of the heart is drastically reduced by blockage of one or more of the coronary arteries. This is one of the principal reasons for devising strategies to limit infarct size. But another lesson being learned, according to Leonard Cobb of Harborview Medical Center in Seattle, is that many persons who experience ventricular fibrillation show no evidence of a recent infarct. Cobb, who is medical director of Medic I, a Seattle community program for delivering emergency medical aid outside the hospital, says that this is true for more than half of those resuscitated in their program. However, most of the patients do have dead cardiac tissue as a result of heart attacks that occurred months or years earlier. And the coronary arteries of almost all are blocked sufficiently to reduce the supply of blood and oxygen to the heart even though tissue may not actually have been killed.

A larger double-blind study, including more than 3000 heart attack patients randomized between the control and treated groups, was conducted in 67 hospital centers, most of which were in Great Britain. The results of the study, which was coordinated by K. G. Green of Imperial Chemical Industries, Ltd., in Alderley Park, Great Britain, showed that there were fewer sudden deaths among patients treated with practolol than among controls (the numbers were 30 and 52, respectively); moreover, there were fewer cardiac deaths of all kinds in the treated group during the 12 months the patients were followed. However, the side effects produced by practolol were serious enough that the physicians conducting the trial considered this drug to be unsuitable for long-term use. They recommended that it be replaced by other drugs with similar mechanisms of action.

Practolol and alprenolol are β-blocking agents; they block the transmission of the sympathetic nerve impulses that increase the heart's irritability. Propranolol, the only β-blocker approved by the Food and Drug Administration (FDA) for use in the United States for treating cardiac arrhythmias, is one of three antiarrhythmic drugs most commonly prescribed here. The other two are procaine amide and quinidine. In addition, the drug lidocaine is usually used in hospitals but must be administered intravenously and is not suitable for outpatient therapy.

None of these agents is ideal. All cause side effects, including weakness, dizziness, nausea, vomiting, diarrhea, or reactions similar to those produced by allergies. And many patients do not respond to any of these drugs. In one study, Bernard Lown and his colleagues at the Harvard School of Public Health found that procaine amide and quinidine controlled the arrhythmias of only about one-quarter of the patients taking them.

One problem is that the doses required to produce therapeutic benefits are only slightly lower than those that produce toxic effects. Many people cannot tolerate doses high enough to do any good. Several investigators expressed concern that so few antiarrhythmic agents are available in this country. They think that the FDA regulations have made it too difficult and expensive for pharmaceutical companies to develop drugs needed by a large number of people.

Nevertheless, three new drugs for controlling arrhythmias, aprindine, disopyramide phosphate, and tocainide, are now undergoing early clinical trials in this country. All have proven effective in a limited number of patients chosen because they had a high frequency of life-threatening arrhythmias that were refractory to the more standard agents.

According to Douglas Zipes of the Indiana University School of Medicine, aprindine reduced the number of ventricular premature beats experienced by 20 of the 23 patients receiving the drug, but it did not eliminate the abnormal beats in any of the patients. Ventricular premature beats occur when the ventricles contract earlier in the cardiac cycle than they should. The agent did prevent the recurrence of ventricular tachycardia and fibrillation in 19 of the patients. (Here ventricular tachycardia is defined as three or more ventricular premature beats in succession.) There are several kinds of tachycardia, which is usually defined as an abnormally fast heart beat; some of them are not dangerous. But ventricular premature beats and ventricular tachycardia are dangerous arrhythmias that may evolve into fibrillation.

During the study, five of the patients died from heart attacks or heart failure, but none died from ventricular arrhythmias not associated with heart attacks. Zipes said that several patients experienced neurological side effects, including tremor, dizziness, hallucinations, and loss of movements, at the higher doses given. Reducing the dosage eliminated the side effects (except the tremor) but not the therapeutic benefits in all the patients who continued on the drug. Only one had to stop taking it.

In a study of 15 patients with intractable arrhythmias, Donald Harrison and his colleagues at Stanford University School of Medicine found that tocainide suppressed the ventricular premature beats of 11 patients. The incidence of the beats was reduced by 90 percent at doses not associated with side effects. The patients served as their own controls, first receiving the placebo and then the drug in a single-blind study.

Harrison says that one of the advantages of tocainide is that the agent is relatively long-lasting and need be taken only two or three times daily. Because the commonly used drugs are rapidly eliminated from the body, patients have to take them every 4 to 6 hours, including during the night, in order to maintain effective therapeutic concentrations in the blood and avoid toxic doses.

Disopyramide phosphate is a third experimental antiarrhythmic drug now being studied by a few investigators including Bernard Tabatznik of Sinai Hospital of Baltimore and Leonard Dreifus of the Lankenau Hospital in Lancaster, Pennsylvania. Tabatznik has found that the drug will eliminate or reduce by 90 percent the incidence of a number of different arrhythmias. The duration of the experiment was short, only a few hours for most of the patients, but a few with serious arrhythmias have been maintained on the drug for up to 2 years.

The mechanisms by which the newer agents act are still under investigation and, like those of the older ones, not completely understood. The beating of the heart is normally regulated by an intrinsic pacemaker, a small strip of tissue called the sinoatrial node, located in the right atrium (the atria are the small upper chambers of the heart) near the spot where the blood enters the heart from the veins. The sinoatrial node automatically sends out rhythmic electrical signals that stimulate the atria to contract and that then spread through a specialized conduction pathway to trigger contraction in the ventricles.

The same pathway also participates in the transmission of abnormal signals, which may originate in or around dead or ischemic tissue, that sometimes culminate in ventricular fibrillation. In one way or another, all of the drugs act on the cells in the conduction pathway to make it more difficult for aberrant impulses to enter the path and be transmitted throughout the ventricles. Some of the drugs act directly on the conducting cells; propranolol and the other β-blockers suppress the pathway indirectly by inhibiting the transmission of excitatory signals from sympathetic neurons, but they may, at high concentrations, also have a direct effect.

Many investigators think that the heart tissue becomes electrically unstable as a result of the ischemia of coronary heart disease and that this instability predisposes the heart to dangerous arrhythmias. Lown defines electrical instability as the condition in which a stimulus of threshold intensity (on average, the lowest that will produce a response), which ordinarily produces only a single response, induces repetitive activity in cardiac muscle. A stimulus substantially above threshold is needed to cause repetitive activity in the normal heart. Although the required intensity is lower for the infarcted heart, it is still above threshold.

Lown and his colleagues have developed a technique for assessing the electrical stability of the hearts of laboratory animals, usually dogs in their experiments. They showed that 2 minutes after tying off a coronary artery the threshold for producing ventricular fibrillation dropped markedly; it returned to normal within 5 minutes. Lown says that these changes paralleled the emergence and recession of arrhythmias.

Lown thinks that, although the electrical instability predisposes to malignant arrhythmias, the precipitation of ventricular fibrillation probably depends on additional factors, such as stress acting through the sympathetic nervous system. The Harvard investigators showed that stimulating a particular brain center reduced the threshold for electrically induced fibrillation in dogs without occlusions but did not spontaneously elicit arrhythmias. However, stimulation of the brain center produced a tenfold increase in the incidence of spontaneous ventricular fibrillation in dogs with occluded coronary arteries. Experiments with inhibitors of the activity of sympathetic neurons indicated that these changes were mediated by this branch of the autonomic nervous system. Direct stimulation of sympathetic nerve cells also lowered the threshold for ventricular fibrillation.

In order to examine the effects of stress itself on the threshold for ventricular fibrillation, the Harvard investigators suspended the dogs in slings, a situation in which the dogs manifested their stress by a number of physiological symptoms, including increased salivation, restlessness, and an elevated heart rate. According to Lown, the threshold was signifiantly lower when the dogs were in the slings than when they were left undisturbed in comfortable cages.

As further evidence that stress and the activity of the sympathetic nervous system predispose to dangerous arrhythmias, Lown cites experiments in which the investigators found that the number and severity of ventricular premature beats of 21 of 26 patients with coronary heart disease were reduced during sleep. The five who either had no decrease or an increase (one case) were the only patients in the study who had taken sleeping pills, although the significance of this observation is unclear. Lown thinks that the reduction is due to the decline in sympathetic activity that occurs during sleep.

For some of the patients, sleep was more effective than drugs, including propranolol, in reducing their arrhythmias, even though part of propranolol's action is thought to be the result of its blocking sympathetic activity on the heart. Lown thinks that the results indicate that the neurological trigger for the arrhythmias may be a more appropriate target for drug therapy than the heart itself.

The use of surgery to prevent certain types of arrhythmias is also being explored, especially for individuals with a severe form of the Wolff-Parkinson-White syndrome. Persons with this syndrome have one or more abnormal pathways, in addition to the normal one, for conducting contraction impulses from the atria to the ventricles. Many persons with this syndrome have no symptoms and may even be unaware that they have it. A few, however, have frequent and prolonged bouts of very fast heartbeats that may be disabling, life-threatening, and unresponsive to drug therapy. According to John Gallagher and surgeon Will Sealy of the Duke University Medical Center, it is possible to identify the abnormal pathway in these patients and interrupt it surgically. They performed the operation on 78 patients by the end of 1976. Seventy-five of the patients survived, and 71 no longer have symptoms.

A development by the Duke group that often facilitates the surgery for Wolff-Parkinson-White syndrome and may permit surgical treatment for other intractable arrhythmias is the use of a cryogenic probe to destroy the abnormal pathway by freezing it. Gallagher says that, when the tissue to be killed is located on the exterior of the heart, the freezing procedure can be carried out without stopping the heart and putting the patient on the heart-lung machine. This makes the operation much simpler and greatly lowers its risks. One 9-year-old boy underwent such surgery and was able to go home 7 days later.

Surgeon Robert Anderson and Gallagher are exploring the possibility that cryogenic surgery can benefit patients with certain other intractable arrhythmias, but Gallagher points out that, whereas surgery may be the optimum therapy for some patients severely afflicted by the Wolff-Parkinson-White syndrome, it will probably be the last resort for most other types of patients.

Another strategy for preventing life-threatening arrhythmias involves the use of pacemakers. The devices are often used to accelerate slow heart rates. Several investigators are now attempting to use the devices to abrogate the electrical signals that give rise to ventricular tachycardia and fibrillation. The devices developed thus far require the patients to turn them on when they feel the heart beating arrhythmically. The next step is to develop a computer-controlled device that can detect the signal and interrupt it automatically.

Because of the side effects of the drugs currently used, cardiologists do not want to prescribe them for all patients with coronary

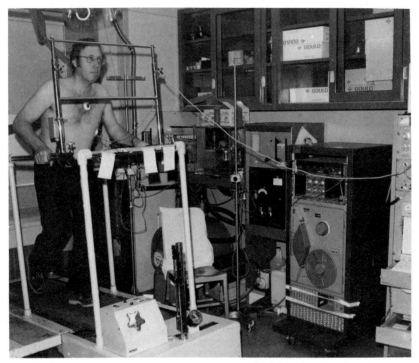

Figure 23. Individual undergoing a stress electrocardiogram. Electrodes are fastened to the subject's chest with suction cups to record the electrical activity of his heart while he exercises by walking the treadmill. [Source: National Heart, Lung, and Blood Institute]

heart disease. Instead, they want to identify those persons at high risk of sudden death from ventricular fibrillation for whom the benefits of therapy should outweigh the risks. Equally important are methods for determining whether therapy with a particular drug is working.

Persons who have already survived one episode of cardiac arrest are known to be at high risk because many suffer additional episodes within a relatively short time. But practically all heart attack victims or individuals with coronary heart disease have occasional ventricular premature beats if their hearts are monitored for long periods of time. Thus, the mere presence or absence of the beats has little prognostic significance. However, most cardiologists think that characteristics of the beats, including their frequency, whether or not

CONTROL

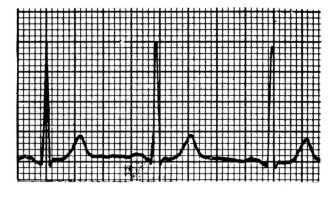

5 MIN. EXERCISE

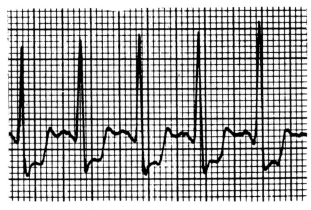

Figure 24. Electrocardiograms (ECG's) taken at rest and during exercise. The upper tracing shows a normal, resting ECG. The lower tracing shows an abnormal ECG recorded during exercise. The segment of the ECG immediately following the sharp peak is markedly depressed. This change indicates that the heart muscle is not receiving an adequate blood flow during exercise. [Source: National Heart, Lung, and Blood Institute]

they occur in sequences, and their position in the cardiac cycle, determine the severity of the irregularities and can be useful in determining a patient's prognosis.

The detection methods most commonly used are the stress electrocardiogram (ECG) and 12- or 24-hour monitoring by means of a lightweight recording electrocardiograph worn by the patients. The biggest advantage that stress ECG's have over extended monitoring is that the former can be done quickly and relatively few heartbeats need to be analyzed. During the course of 24 hours the heart beats about 100,000 times. However, investigators, including Jerome Cox at Washington University School of Medicine and John Fitzgerald at Stanford, are developing techniques for automatically scanning the long records or condensing them by means of computer-assisted devices that only record when the arrhythmias occur.

The idea behind stress testing is that the applied stress, usually exercise such as walking a treadmill (Figures 23 and 24), may cause the heart of a person with coronary artery disease to become deficient in oxygen, with the result that the number of arrhythmic beats is increased. For example, Lown and his colleagues found that exercise increased the number of ventricular premature beats threefold in men with coronary artery disease and increased the frequency of ventricular tachycardia almost eight times in a 3-minute period.

The biggest disadvantage of the stress ECG is that there is a chance that the patient may go into cardiac arrest during the test or shortly thereafter. Despite this danger, numerous investigators have had extensive experience with exercise testing and there have been few fatal complications. Paul Rochmis of Fairfax, Virginia, and Henry Blackburn of the University of Minnesota reviewed 170,000 tests conducted at 73 clinical centers and found only 16 deaths within 24 hours after completion of the ECG.

Thus, there are safe techniques for detecting dangerous arrhythmias and predicting which patients are most likely to experience ventricular fibrillation. The most pressing need is the development of therapeutic regimens for controlling the arrhythmias without inflicting unacceptable side effects on the individuals undergoing them. Cardiologists hope that the investigations now under way may help to fill that need.

16

CORONARY BYPASS SURGERY
Debate Over Its Benefits

Cardiologists are becoming more and more adept at diagnosing coronary artery disease. But once they find that a person's coronary arteries are obstructed, they may be faced with a dilemma about what sort of treatment to prescribe. Many recommend coronary bypass surgery – a procedure in which a vein from a patient's leg is grafted onto the clogged coronary artery to shunt blood past the obstruction into the heart. (Figure 25). Others are very cautious about endorsing this procedure and believe drugs may provide benefits comparable to those of surgery.

Despite its controversial status, coronary bypass surgery has become a big business in the United States. According to Richard Ross of Johns Hopkins University, about 25,000 such operations were performed in 1971 and, by 1973, this number had doubled. He estimates that at least 65,000 operations were performed last year and that each cost at least $10,000. (This price includes the surgeon's fee and charges for hospitalization, laboratory tests, equipment, and medical care.) Thus, about $650 million was spent on coronary bypass operations last year. In contrast, the total budget of the National Heart, Lung, and Blood Institute was only $400 million.

In recent years, bypass surgery has become commonplace at many community hospitals, but most of the operations are performed at teaching hospitals and medical centers such as the Cleveland Clinic, the Texas Heart Institute in Houston, and the Mayo Clinic in Rochester, Minnesota. For example, 2,700 operations were performed at the Cleveland Clinic last year and 12,000 were performed there in

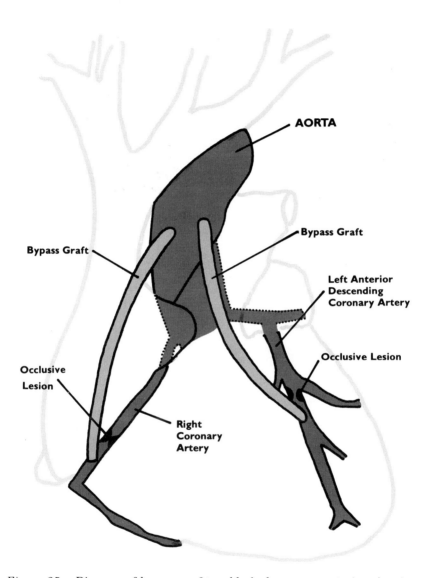

Figure 25. Diagram of bypasses of two blocked coronary arteries. A vein from the leg is used to divert blood past the occluded arteries.

the past decade, according to Donald Effler, who was formerly at the Cleveland Clinic and is now at Saint Joseph's Hospital in Syracuse, New York.

Most patients who have had this operation are extremely enthusiastic about it, as are many surgeons who perform it and cardiologists who recommend it. Effler, Mason Sones of the Cleveland Clinic, Denton Cooley of the Texas Heart Institute, and other proponents of the operation state unequivocally that it relieves symptoms of coronary artery disease and prolongs lives. Some cardiologists recommend this operation even for asymptomatic patients with coronary artery disease. A number of other investigators, however, are asking whether the operation actually improves blood flow to the heart and whether people treated with surgery do live longer than those treated with drugs.

To assess the results of coronary bypass surgery, investigators have looked at changes in blood flow to the heart after the operation. A common way to determine blood flow in coronary arteries is to use contrast angiography. In this procedure, a catheter is inserted into the patient's heart, a radiopaque medium is injected, and x-ray pictures of the coronary arteries are made.

Lawrence Griffith, Stephen Achuff, and their associates at the Johns Hopkins University Medical School used contrast angiography to determine that a significant number of occlusions occur in coronary arteries after bypass surgery, thus impeding blood flow. This result was confirmed by six other groups of researchers. Specifically, the Hopkins group compared patients' coronary arteries before surgery to their arteries 6 months after surgery and found that 40 percent of the arteries had new occlusions. These investigators also looked at the arteries of a group of patients who were not operated on. Only 6 percent of the arteries of this control group had new occlusions after 6 months.

Most of the new occlusions that followed surgery were in the bypassed artery and were upstream from the graft (between the point of narrowing in the coronary artery and the point of attachment of the graft). This is less significant than if they were downstream, but it still means that the blood supply to the heart becomes dependent on the grafted vessel remaining open. This may affect only a small proportion of patients since most grafts do remain open. Floyd Loop and his associates at the Cleveland Clinic found that 83 percent of

185 grafts were open 4 years or more after surgery. For those few patients whose grafts close, new occlusions in the bypassed arteries may cause irreversible damage to heart muscle.

Although most people with angina pectoris obtain symptomatic relief immediately after surgery, this relief may not continue indefinitely. E. L. Alderman and his associates at Stanford University School of Medicine found that 40 percent of 350 patients who had angina pectoris and who had this operation had a recurrence or worsening of their chest pain within 2 to 5 years after surgery. These investigators also reported that the chest pains of a small number of patients lessened with time but that a significant fraction of these people developed infarctions, or dead areas of heart muscle, before their pain disappeared.

Relief of pain just after bypass surgery may not necessarily be due to improved coronary circulation. Other explanations are also possible. For example, new infarctions may occur during or just after the surgery and may deaden the heart muscle that had been causing the pain.

Many cardiologists believe that only a small percentage of patients have new infarctions immediately after bypass surgery, but this belief was recently questioned by Melvin Platt, James Willerson, Frederick Bonte, and their associates at the University of Texas Health Center at Dallas. In order to detect new infarctions, these researchers injected patients with a radionuclide tracer that lodges in recently damaged heart muscle. The damaged tissue can then be seen because the radionuclide emits γ-rays that can be detected with a scintillation camera. Platt and his associates studied 48 patients between 3 and 5 days after surgery. They found evidence of newly damaged heart muscle in 15 patients (31 percent). In contrast, when they looked for damage with electrocardiograms or with analyses of two enzymes that appear in the blood when heart muscle dies, they found new damage in only 6 of these patients (12 percent). Electrocardiograms and the presence of these enzymes are the techniques most often used to determine whether new infarctions occur after bypass surgery. Incidences of new infarctions may vary from hospital to hospital, however. Loop reports that only 4 percent of patients at the Cleveland Clinic have postoperative infarctions as measured by enzymes, electrocardiograms, and also by angiography, which is more accurate than these other two methods.

Another explanation for the immediate postsurgical relief of angina is that surgery acts as a placebo. Ross has described an example of how powerful such a placebo effect can be. About 20 years ago, it was commonplace to ligate patients' internal mammary arteries in order to relieve their angina pectoris. The operation achieved this purpose, but, in 1959, an experiment was performed to determine whether there was a physiological reason for the pain relief. (For ethical reasons, this experiment could not be performed today.) Patients with angina pectoris were randomly divided into two groups. Those in one group had their internal mammary arteries ligated. Those in the other group underwent sham operations. About 70 percent of the patients from each group had no angina following their surgery. Members of both groups had improved performance as measured by exercise electrocardiograms. Some investigators object to this example of placebo effects. Loop, for example, claims that placebo effects of sham operations tend to wane by 6 months after surgery and are almost always gone by 1 year. Relief of pain following bypass surgery, however, generally lasts for years.

Despite these questions about why coronary bypass surgery relieves pain, most cardiologists recommend it for patients with severe angina pectoris that is not relieved when the people are given drugs such as nitrates and propranolol. Sones, however, does not think that this is a valid criterion. He points out that a physician's recognition of the kind of pain a person suffers is limited by the person's ability to describe it. And the patient's perceptions of pain can be greatly affected by emotional stress. According to Sones, as many as 25 percent of the people who are referred to the Cleveland Clinic because they have chest pains and who are being treated by their referring physicians for coronary artery disease turn out not to have occluded coronary arteries. Sones advocates coronary bypass surgery for people with significantly occluded coronary arteries independently of whether they have angina pectoris. The operation, he contends, will prolong these peoples' lives.

Sones, Effler, and others are so convinced that coronary bypass surgery prolongs lives in comparison to medical treatment that they believe randomized controlled clinical trials of the effects of this operation on mortality rates are unethical. Sones believes that people could not possibly give informed consent to enter a randomized trial. Anyone who does give consent cannot be adequately informed, he says. Nonetheless, a number of randomized trials are being conducted. Those conducting the trials are as convinced that the question of whether coronary bypass surgery prolongs lives when compared to medical treatment is still open as Sones and others are that it is not.

Evidence that coronary bypass surgery prolongs lives comes from studies of patients who were not assigned treatment at random. For example, in one often-cited study, William Sheldon and his associates at the Cleveland Clinic compared the mortality rates of 1000 people who had this operation at the clinic to those of 469 people who were diagnosed at the clinic as having coronary artery disease but were not operated on. These controls were all diagnosed between 1960 and 1965, which is before the bypass operation was developed. Those patients who were diagnosed between 1960 and 1965 and who subsequently underwent the operation were excluded from the control group. The average mortality per year in the surgical group was 3.3 percent. In the nonsurgical group it was 8.8 percent.

Many investigators are unconvinced by results of studies, such as the Cleveland Clinic study, in which "historical controls" are used. They point out that the patients studied in the past are not necessarily comparable to those studied more recently. Means of diagnosis change, supportive care changes, and random changes can occur with time in the type of patients admitted to an institution such as the Cleveland Clinic. In addition, several investigators, such as Robert Rosati of Duke University and Richard Kronmal of the University of Washington believe that there is a bias in the Cleveland Clinic data that derives from the way the historical controls were selected. Since patients who were diagnosed between 1960 and 1965 and who subsequently had bypass surgery when it was introduced were eliminated from the control group, the control group may have had an artificially high proportion of people who died before bypass surgery was introduced or who were too sick to undergo the operation.

Loop contends that this bias did not occur in the selection of the control group. Only a few patients were eliminated from the control group because they subsequently had the vein bypass operation, he says. Further support comes from similar studies with historical controls at other institutions, such as the Texas Heart Institute, which also indicate that the surgical patients may live longer than those who did not have the operation.

Thomas Killip of Northwestern University Medical School points out that the use of historical controls is justified only if there is no change in the treatment of the control group. But about 5 years ago drugs such as propranolol were introduced to treat people with angina pectoris. These drugs reduce the response of the heart to stress and thereby may prevent the occurrence of irreversible damage to the hearts of people with angina pectoris. Killip believes that these new drugs make it equally likely that lives would be prolonged with medical as with surgical treatments.

Rosati and his associates are conducting a nonrandomized trial that compares surgery to medical treatment and that avoids some of these problems with historical controls. The trial participants are people with coronary artery disease who were diagnosed at Duke University Medical Center between 1969 and 1974 and whose treatments were prescribed by their individual physicians. Thus the medical and surgical groups were diagnosed and treated during the same time period. The assumption is that, as a group, physicians decide between medical and surgical treatment at random. Rosati and his colleagues followed 490 people who underwent the operation and 611 who did not. They conclude that surgery did not affect the mortality rates of these groups.

Several large-scale randomized trials are under way, but among them only the Veterans Administration (VA) trial has continued long enough for results to be published. The VA Cooperative Study began in 1970 and includes patients at 13 VA hospitals. So far, 1015 people with angina pectoris have been randomly assigned medical or surgical treatment. For the VA patients as a whole, there are as yet no statistically significant differences in mortality rates of the medical and surgical groups. The VA is, however, looking at subgroups of patients to see if any differences in mortality rates can be discerned.

Of particular interest, because many investigators believe the preliminary data are promising, are patients whose left main coronary arteries are at least 50 percent occluded. The left main coronary artery branches before it reaches the heart, and the two branches supply blood to a large area of heart muscle. Thus extensive coronary damage can result from blockage of this artery. Of the 1015 VA patients, 113 had this artery occluded. According to Timothy Takaro of the VA Hospital in Asheville, North Carolina, the mortality rate of the surgical patients in this subgroup is lower than that of the medical patients at 18, 25, and 30 months after entry into the study. This difference is statistically significant, Takaro claims. At 36 months, however, the number of survivors in the medical and surgical groups was so small that the differences between the two groups became statistically insignificant. Nonetheless, many cardiologists say they are sufficiently convinced by these preliminary results to recommend surgery for people with diseased left main coronary arteries.

Two randomized, controlled clinical trials of surgical and medical treatments are being conducted by the NHLBI. One of these, the Coronary Artery Surgery Trial (CAST) includes people who have demonstrable coronary artery disease and who satisfy specific clinical criteria. For example, people who have chest pain when they walk a block or climb a flight of stairs but have no pain at rest are eligible. People with more severe angina pectoris are not. The hope is that these clinical criteria will ensure a relatively homogeneous group of subjects for the study and facilitate interpretation of the results. Recruitment for CAST should be completed by January 1978; between 800 and 1000 patients are anticipated. Mortality rates will be determined during a period of 5 years. In addition, the NHLBI investigators plan to study how the participants feel after medical or surgical treatment by asking them questions about the quality of their lives.

The second NHLBI clinical trial involves people with unstable angina pectoris. The designers of this trial define unstable angina in two ways. First, it can mean angina pectoris that is of recent onset either at rest or on exertion. Alternatively, it can mean angina pectoris that had previously occurred in predictable circumstances – after climbing two flights of stairs, say. If this angina suddenly begins to occur under different circumstances – climbing one flight of stairs, for example – the NHLBI group defines it as unstable angina pectoris. Unstable angina pectoris has been thought to signal an imminent threat to patients' lives, and many cardiologists have advised emergency coronary bypass surgery. Preliminary results of the NHLBI trial indicate that the prognosis for people with unstable angina pectoris is not necessarily so grave.

Recruitment for the NHLBI study of unstable angina pectoris began in August 1972 and is still continuing. According to Peter Frommer of the NHLBI, about 280 people have been recruited so far, and recruitment will end when 300 are recruited. The follow-up time for this trial is something of a problem. When the trial was designed, unstable angina pectoris was thought to be such a serious condition that 1 year would be sufficient to determine whether medical or surgical treatments affected mortality rates. This turned out to be inadequate, and the question of the length of the follow-up period is now under study.

One of the aims of the randomized trial of treatments of unstable angina pectoris is to identify subsets of patients with high risk compared to others with this condition. Some investigators, however, think that the ongoing clinical trials are likely to yield convincing data on long-term survival rates only when the trial participants are considered as a whole and not when they are broken down into subsets on the basis of specific diagnostic criteria. This makes it difficult to determine who will benefit from the surgery. Cardiologists can always argue that their patients are individuals and they must prescribe for their patients as individuals and not on the basis of the average behavior of a large group of trial participants. And patients with coronary artery disease are likely to be receptive to the suggestion that, for them, this surgery will be of benefit. As Effler points out, patients even now go to the Cleveland Clinic, where cardiologists are enthusiastic about bypass surgery, rather than to institutions where cardiologists are more hesitant to endorse this procedure.

Some cardiologists who advocate this surgery argue that the ongoing clinical trials cannot determine whether surgery can prolong lives when compared to medical treatment. The problem, they say, is that the current success and popularity of the surgery make it hard to design a good clinical trial. These advocates of surgery claim that institutions where surgery is good and whose patients have low mortality rates are unwilling to participate in randomized clinical trials. The ongoing trials may thereby yield misleadingly poor results of surgery. Thus results from current research on the question of whether coronary bypass surgery prolongs lives in comparison to medical treatment may not settle the debate over this question.

17

THE AGING HEART
Changes in Function and Response to Drugs

Most studies of heart disease have been concerned with heart disease in those under 65 — the so-called "premature" heart disease. This emphasis is understandable both because premature heart disease strikes people who are more likely to be economically productive and because it usually is more shocking to see a younger than an older person die or become disabled. But the fact remains that most heart disease occurs among people aged 65 or older. Heart disease is so common among old people that it accounts for more than 40 percent of the deaths in this age group.

Heart disease in old people may have different causes and require different treatment than premature heart disease. The changes in the heart that come with age are likely to affect its susceptibility to damage and its response to drugs. In order to determine the degree to which conclusions from data on premature heart disease can be generalized to older people, investigators are studying the epidemiology of heart disease in the elderly and the biochemical changes that occur in the aging heart.

It would be desirable to study the effects of aging on the cardiovascular system by recording physiological changes that occur in members of a group of people as they relate to their chances of dying from heart disease over the course of their adult lives. This is not often done because it is expensive and because people tend to drop out of long-term studies. Thus, only a few studies of this type are being conducted, including the U.S. Public Health Service's Framingham Study.

In 1949, the USPHS began recruiting about 6000 people between the ages of 30 and 59 from the town of Framingham, Massachusetts. This continuing investigation is providing some insights into the effects of risk factors for heart disease on people of all ages, including those over the age of 65.

According to William Kannel, who directs the Framingham Study, some major risk factors in younger people do not seem to affect the elderly. Serum cholesterol concentrations and cigarette smoking, for example, are not good predictors of heart attacks or strokes in the elderly. (Smoking is associated with the development of lung cancer and emphysema in the elderly, however.) And diabetes seems to have less effect on old men than young, although it does predispose old women to develop heart disease. Kannel says that the best predictors of heart disease in old people are hypertension, electrocardiogram findings, high-density lipoproteins (which are associated with lowered risks) and, in women, diabetes. He emphasizes that, contrary to a widespread belief, hypertension is as much a threat to the old as to the young. The lower an old person's blood pressure, the lower his or her risk of developing heart disease. (Old women with low blood pressure, Kannel says, are "practically immortal.")

Since risk factors for heart disease in the young may not be risk factors for the elderly, not all research on the causes of premature heart disease may be applicable to heart disease in old people. In order to understand the genesis of heart disease in the elderly, it is helpful to know both the biochemical and the physiological changes that occur with age. An emphasis on studies of both physiology and biochemistry is the thrust of research at the National Institute of Aging (NIA) in Baltimore, where investigators are now beginning to piece together a picture of changes in the aging heart.

One of the most striking physiological changes that occurs with age is a decline in the heart's ability to respond to stress. This decline, first reported as early as 1929, has been confirmed by numerous investigators. During the stress of exercise, heart rate and blood flow increase, but the magnitude of these increases is smaller in older than in younger people.

James Conway of Imperial Chemicals in Cheshire, England, and his associates find that these age differences in response to stress are obliterated when younger people are given propranolol. Propranolol blocks the response of the heart to catecholamines — agents that are secreted in response to stress. Catecholamines bind to specific receptors on heart cells and cause the heart to beat faster and increase the strength of its contractions. Propranolol prevents the binding of catecholamines.

Conway's result indicates either that old people secrete fewer catecholamines in response to stress or that their hearts respond less well to them. Edward Lakatta of the NIA reports evidence that supports the latter explanation. He and his associates found that the responses of people, rats, and dogs to catecholamines all diminish with age.

In order to study the basis of this decreased response to catecholamines, Lakatta and his associates, together with Myron Weisfeldt of Johns Hopkins University Medical School, isolated heart muscle from old and young rats and compared the responses of these muscles to catecholamines and calcium. Catecholamines increase the amount of calcium supplied to the contractile proteins of heart muscle cells and thereby cause the muscle to contract. It had been previously shown that heart muscle from young rats is stimulated equally well by both catecholamines and calcium. The muscle from old rats responded as well to calcium as muscle from young hearts but less well to catecholamines. Thus the effect of aging seems to be in the ability of catecholamines to affect the release of calcium rather than in the response to calcium per se.

Investigators at the NIA find that there is an age-associated decline in the number of catecholamine receptors on heart muscle cells. Isolated heart muscle from both old dogs and old rats has fewer receptors than muscle from young animals. Such a decrease could be a cause of the observed lack of responsiveness. George Roth of the NIA and others believe that diminishing numbers of hormone receptors are a universal characteristic of aging. Such decreases have been shown to occur in cells other than heart cells and to affect receptors for several kinds of hormones.

It is also possible that cardiac receptors for digitalis are lost with age. Digitalis binds to cardiac receptors and increases the strength of contractions. Roth finds that heart muscle from old rats responds poorly to digitalis. If human hearts respond similarly, digitalis may be less effective in old than in young people. Digitalis is commonly used to treat congestive heart failure, but patients who take it may suffer from serious side effects. According to Paula Goldberg and Jay Roberts of the Medical College of Pennsylvania in Philadelphia, old people have often been reported to react severely to concentrations of digitalis that do not generally injure younger people. These reactions include cardiac arrhythmias and neurological disturbances.

A second reason for the heart's decreased response to stress with age may be that the heart muscle changes its mechanical and biochemical characteristics. Many investigators have found that contractions are prolonged in hearts of old people and old laboratory animals. A contraction consists of a period during which the heart muscle builds up tension and one in which the tension is released. Harold Spurgeon and his associates at the NIA report that isolated heart muscle from old rats and old dogs relaxes more slowly than muscle from younger animals.

Studies by other investigators have shown that several reasons for the prolonged relaxation period of old heart muscle are possible. In order for heart muscle to relax, calcium must be removed from the contractile proteins and taken up by the sarcoplasmic reticulum, which is a separate compartment in the muscle cell. An increase in relaxation time may be caused by a decrease in the rate of calcium removal by the sarcoplasmic reticulum. Jeffrey Froehlich and his associates at the NIA recently isolated sarcoplasmic reticulum from rat heart muscle. Their preliminary results indicate that the isolated material absorbs calcium less readily as the animal ages.

Froehlich has not ruled out the possibility that other mechanisms of calcium uptake may compensate for these age-associated changes in the sarcoplasmic reticulum. But he does think his results are a first step to discovering why old heart muscle relaxes slowly.

Froehlich and Robert Tomenek of the University of Iowa point out that changes in the sarcoplasmic reticulum could be secondary, rather than primary, effects of aging. Heart muscle tends to hypertrophy with age, and there is some evidence that hypertrophy may be associated with a decrease in the activity of the sarcoplasmic reticulum. This does not necessarily mean that hypertrophy causes this decrease in activity.

Most results on the effects of hypertrophy are based on studies of rat muscle. But these changes also seem to occur in people. Gary Gerstenblith and his associates at the NIA report that human hearts become thicker with age. For example, the left ventricular wall is about 25 percent thicker at age 80 than at age 30.

Although the recent studies of the biochemistry and physiology of the aging heart do not provide direct evidence of why old hearts become damaged, they do indicate that specific changes occur with age. Knowledge of these and other changes may have important implications for drug therapy.

Roberts and Goldberg have been studying the aging heart with an eye to assessing the use of drugs that counter arrhythmias in the elderly. They found that the electrical activity of cardiac pacemaker cells decreases as rats grow old. This decrease in activity occurs in the pacemaker cells in the right atrium, which normally set the rhythm of the heartbeats, and in pacemaker cells in the ventricles, whose activity becomes apparent only when the heart is damaged in such a way that conduction between the atria and ventricles is blocked. When such a blockage occurs, the ventricular pacemaker cells cause the ventricles to beat at their own rate independently of the atria. Roberts and Goldberg speculate that the possible slowing of the electrical activity of human cardiac pacemakers with age may explain why old people are more susceptible to cardiac arrhythmias than young people.

Roberts and Goldberg find that age-associated changes in the pacemaker cells of rats seemed to modify their response to three antiarrhythmic drugs. One of these drugs, quinidine, is often given to people with arrhythmias arising in the atria. These investigators found that the effects of quinidine on the electrical activity of both atrial and ventricular pacemakers of rats decreased with age. Lidocaine, which is given to people with ventricular arrhythmias, also had a decreased effect on the ventricular pacemakers from old rats. But it had a greater effect on the atrial pacemakers as the rats aged. And propranolol, which is thought to act in a way similar to that of quinidine, had the same effect on old as young pacemaker cells from the atrium and from the ventricle of rats.

Goldberg and Roberts point out that old people may have different reactions to drugs than the young for reasons other than changes in their heart cells. The effects of drugs are related to their absorption by the gastrointestinal system, their distribution in the body, and their metabolism. All change with age.

A complete picture of how and why heart disease occurs and how old people with heart disease should be treated cannot emerge until the aging heart is understood in light of age-associated changes in the rest of the body. But the recent studies of the aging heart are providing direction to the study of heart disease in the elderly.

Appendix I

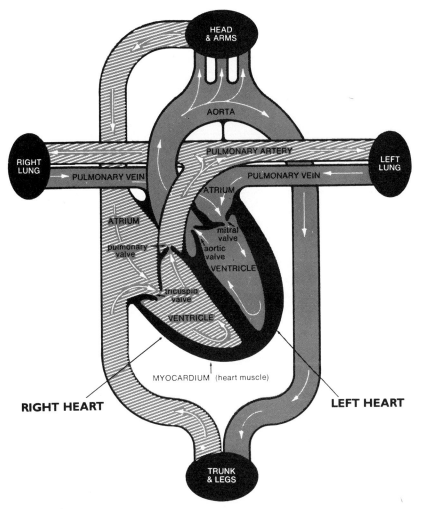

Schematic Diagram of the Heart and Circulatory System

The right heart receives blood from the body and pumps it through the pulmonary artery to the lungs where it picks up oxygen. The blood returns in the pulmonary vein to the left heart. The left heart then pumps the oxygenated blood through the aorta to the body where the oxygen is released for the use of the tissues. [© Reprinted with the permission of the American Heart Association]

Glossary

Italicized words in the definitions are also defined in this glossary.

Adenosine triphosphate (ATP) The major carrier of chemical energy in the cells of all living organisms. Energy trapped in ATP is used to drive energy-requiring reactions; cells will die unless the ATP is constantly replenished.

Adrenalin See *epinephrine*.

Aldosterone A steroid hormone produced by the outer layer (cortex) of the adrenal gland. Aldosterone acts on the kidney to increase retention of sodium ions and water. Because it acts to increase blood volume, the hormone is an important regulator of *blood pressure*.

Alprenolol A drug that is a *β-blocking agent*.

Angina pectoris A condition in which transient chest pains occur, especially during exertion, as a result of partial blockage of the *coronary arteries* and consequent deprivation of an adequate supply of blood and oxygen to a portion of the *heart*.

Angiography See *coronary angiography*.

Angiotensin Angiotensin I, II, and III are peptide hormones that are very potent increasers of *blood pressure*. Overproduction of the hormones may be one cause of *hypertension*.

Angiotensinogen A blood peptide that is split by the action of the *enzyme renin* to produce the *angiotensins*.

Antiarrhythmic agent A drug given to control certain dangerous *cardiac arrhythmias* that may cause *sudden death*.

Aprindine An experimental drug being tested as an *antiarrhythmic agent*.

Arachidonic acid A fatty acid found in many fats and other *lipids* from which several *prostaglandins* are synthesized.

Arrhythmias See *cardiac arrhythmias*.

Arterial endothelium The inner lining of an *artery*.

Arteriole An *artery* of small diameter that branches to form *capillaries*. The state of constriction or dilation of the arterioles is one of the most important determinants of *blood pressure*.

Arteriosclerosis A general term for the condition in which the *arteries* thicken, harden, and lose their elasticity.

Artery Any blood vessel carrying blood away from the *heart*.

Aspirin myocardial infarction study (AMIS) A *clinical trial* to determine whether aspirin protects against recurrent *heart attacks* in patients who have already had at least one.

Atherosclerosis A form of *arteriosclerosis* characterized by the development of *atherosclerotic plaques* in the *arteries*.

Atherosclerotic plaque An abnormal area in the arterial lining that is composed of smooth muscle cells; *lipids,* especially *cholesterol*; and calcium. The plaques may grow until they completely block the *artery*.

Atria The two smaller, upper chambers of the *heart* to which blood returns from the lungs and the rest of the body.

Autonomic nervous system The nervous system that controls functions, such as respiration, blood flow, and the beating of the *heart,* that are not normally under voluntary control.

Baroreceptors Receptors, present in certain major *arteries,* that are activated by an increase in *blood pressure*. Impulses from the baroreceptors signal the brain and *sympathetic nervous system* to lower the *blood pressure*.

β-blocking agent A drug that blocks the transmission of some kinds of impulses from the *sympathetic nervous system*. Some of these agents are used to control *cardiac arrhythmias* or high *blood pressure*.

Blood clot A solidified mass of blood cells, *platelets,* and blood proteins. A clot is normally formed to prevent blood loss when a vessel is cut, but clots may form abnormally in intact blood vessels and clog them.

Blood pressure The pressure of the blood in the *arteries*. It is represented by two figures (120/80, for example). The higher figure represents the pressure (in millimeters of mercury) during *systole* and the lower is that during *diastole*.

Bradykinin See *kinins*.

Capillaries Extremely small blood vessels connecting the *arteries* with the *veins*. Exchange of nutrients and wastes between the blood and tissues takes place in the capillaries.

Cardiac arrest Cessation of the *heart's* beating, often as a result of *ventricular fibrillation*.

Cardiac arrhythmias Disturbances in the normal pattern of the *heart's* beating. Some are not dangerous, but others may lead to *ventricular fibrillation* and *sudden death* if not controlled.

Cardiopulmonary resuscitation (CPR) A technique to restore the circulation of oxygenated blood to all parts of the body of someone whose *heart* has stopped beating. CPR includes mouth-to-mouth resuscitation and external heart massage (exerting firm rhythmic pressure on the chest over the heart).

Cardiovascular disease Disease of the *heart* or blood vessels.

Catecholamine Any one of a group of physiologically active compounds, including the hormones *epinephrine* and *norepinephrine* (also called adrenalin and noradrenalin) produced by the interior portion (medulla) of the adrenal gland and a number of nerve endings. Some of the compounds have profound effects on the *heart* and circulatory system.

Cholesterol A *lipid* (and sterol) which is used by the body as a building block for cellular membranes and for the synthesis of steroid hormones. But it is also a prominent component of *atherosclerotic plaques* and may be involved in the etiology of *atherosclerosis* and *heart* disease.

Chylomicrons Small globules of *lipids* coated with protein; they are the first *lipoproteins* formed when lipids are absorbed from the intestine.

Clinical trial A study in which the efficacy of an experimental preventive or curative treatment for a disease is assessed in human subjects.

Collateral arteries Small *arteries* branching from the main *coronary arteries* and carrying blood to the *heart* muscle. When a coronary artery is blocked, additional collateral arteries may form to the portion of heart muscle that was deprived of a blood supply.

Computerized axial tomography (CAT) A computerized method for constructing a three-dimensional view of an organ from two-dimensional images (usually x-ray images) taken from several angles.

Congenital defect   Any defect present at birth.

Congestive heart failure   Weakening of the *heart* accompanied by the accumulation of fluid in the abdomen, legs, and lungs as a result of the heart's inability to pump blood at its normal capacity.

Coronary angiography   An x-ray technique that enables the clinician to visualize the *heart* and *coronary arteries* and assess their function.

Coronary artery   Either of two arteries that carry blood to the *heart* muscle itself. (As it leaves the aorta, the left coronary artery divides almost immediately into two large branches, so that there are effectively three coronary arteries.)

Coronary artery disease   A condition in which any of the *coronary arteries* become partially or completely blocked with *atherosclerotic plaques*. *Angina pectoris* or a *heart attack* may result.

Coronary artery surgery trial (CAST)   A *clinical trial* in which *coronary bypass surgery* is being compared to nonsurgical therapies for *coronary artery disease*.

Coronary bypass surgery   Surgery in which a *vein,* often from the leg, is grafted onto a clogged *coronary artery* to shunt blood past the obstruction to the *heart* muscle.

Coronary care unit (CCU)   A specialized hospital unit in which *heart* patients are carefully monitored for heart irregularities and immediately treated if they occur.

Coronary drug project   A *clinical trial* designed to determine whether *cholesterol*-lowering drugs would decrease the recurrence of *heart attacks* in men who had already had at least one.

Coronary heart disease   The same as *coronary artery disease*.

Coronary occlusion   Blockage of a *coronary artery*; frequently used as a synonym for *heart attack*.

Coronary thrombosis   Blockage of a *coronary artery* with a type of *blood clot*; a synonym for *heart attack*.

Creatine phosphokinase (CPK)   An *enzyme* released into the blood from dead *heart* muscle. Measurement of its concentration in blood is used to help diagnose *heart attacks* and measure *infarct* size.

Diastole The portion of the heartbeat between contractions (*systoles*) when the *heart* muscle relaxes and the heart fills with blood.

Digitalis A drug often given to persons with *heart failure* to strengthen the beating of their *hearts*.

Disopyramide phosphate An experimental *antiarrhythmic agent*.

Diuretic A drug used to increase excretion of water by the kidneys. Diuretics are frequently used to treat *congestive heart failure* and *hypertension*.

Double-blind study A *clinical trial* in which neither the patients nor the physicians know who is receiving the test drug and who is receiving a *placebo*.

Ejection fraction The percentage of blood ejected from the *heart* in a single beat.

Electrocardiogram (ECG) A tracing showing the electrical activity of the *heart* during the contraction cycle. Abnormalities in the tracing can be used to diagnose *cardiac arrhythmias* and *heart attacks*.

Emission tomography A variation of *tomography* in which the organ to be visualized is specifically labeled with a radioactive material and two-dimensional images are made of the labeled organs from several angles.

Endoperoxides These highly unstable *prostaglandins* (designated PGG_2 and PGH_2) are key intermediates in the synthesis of several other prostaglandins and the *thromboxanes*.

Enzyme A biological catalyst that greatly increases the rate of a biochemical reaction. Enzymes are proteins.

Epidemiology The science of investigating the causes of a disease by seeking to identify the conditions and characteristics associated with the development of the disease in different populations.

Epinephrine One of the *catecholamines*. Released by sympathetic nerve terminals to the *heart*, it greatly stimulates the beating of that organ.

Essential hypertension *Hypertension* of unknown origin.

Familial hypercholesteremia *Hypercholesteremia* of genetic origin. Persons with the disease may have extremely high concentrations of blood *cholesterol* and severe *atherosclerosis*.

Framingham Study A *prospective study* conducted in Framingham, Massachusetts, that has provided a great deal of information about the *risk factors* for *cardiovascular diseases* as well as other diseases.

Heart The muscular organ that pumps blood to all parts of the body. In mammals, including humans, it is composed of four chambers, two *atria* and two *ventricles*.

Heart attack Damage to the *heart* that occurs when any of the *coronary arteries* are blocked, and the supply of blood to a portion of the heart muscle is interrupted. *Cardiac arrest* may be considered a type of heart attack even though damage to the heart muscle is not always apparent.

Heart failure Condition in which the heart has been so weakened, whether by high *blood pressure, heart attack, rheumatic heart disease,* or birth defects, that it pumps well below its normal capacity.

Heart valve Flaps of tissue that prevent reflux of blood from the *ventricles* to the *atria* or from the pulmonary artery or aorta to the ventricles.

High blood pressure *Hypertension.*

High-density lipoproteins (HDL) *Lipoproteins* that transport *cholesterol* from other tissues to the liver where it may be converted to other compounds or from which it may be excreted into the intestines. High concentrations of HDL appear to be correlated with a lower risk of *heart attacks*.

Historical controls A group of individuals who have had a disease in the past and are used as a control group in a *clinical trial.* The effects of an experimental therapy are assessed by comparing the prognoses of patients given the therapy to those of the historical controls who either had a conventional therapy or no therapy at all.

Hyaluronidase An *enzyme* under investigation as an agent for limiting *infarct* size in *heart attack* victims.

Hypercholesteremia Elevated concentrations of blood *cholesterol,* a condition that may be associated with increased risk of *atherosclerosis* and *heart attack*.

Hypertension Chronically elevated *blood pressures*.

Indomethacin An analgesic drug, related to aspirin, that blocks the synthesis of *prostaglandins* and *thromboxanes*.

Infarct The area of *heart* muscle that is damaged when one or more of the *coronary arteries* supplying blood to the heart is blocked.

Intra-aortic balloon counterpulsation A technique used to increase the *heart's* blood supply. A balloon is inserted into the main *artery* leading out of the heart. The balloon is inflated when the heart is at rest between contractions, which raises the pressure in the arteries and increases the heart's blood supply.

Ischemia A condition in which tissue is not receiving an adequate blood supply.

Isoproterenol A drug sometimes used to treat *heart attack* victims. It increases the amount of blood pumped by the *heart* by increasing contractility and heart rate.

Kallikrein An *enzyme* that produces the *kinins* by catalyzing the splitting of a large peptide found in blood.

Kinins Small peptides that lower the *blood pressure* by increasing secretion of water and sodium ions by the kidney and causing the dilation of blood vessels.

Lidocaine A drug used to treat *cardiac arrhythmias*.

Lipid A substance insoluble in water but soluble in fat solvents, such as alcohol. The *triglycerides* and *cholesterol* are lipids.

Lipid research clinic primary prevention trial A *clinical trial* being conducted by the National Heart, Lung, and Blood Institute and designed to answer the question of whether lowering blood *lipid* concentrations can reduce the incidence of heart disease.

Lipoproteins Complexes of *lipids* and proteins. There are four main types of lipoproteins, classified according to their size and density. The four classes are the *chylomicrons, very-low-density lipoproteins (VLDL), low-density lipoproteins (LDL)*, and *high-density lipoproteins (HDL)*.

Low-density lipoproteins (LDL) The *lipoproteins* that carry most of the *cholesterol* in the blood. Elevated concentrations of LDL have been associated with an increased risk of *heart attacks*.

Lysosomes Membranous sacs inside cells. The lysosomes contain *enzymes* that break down a variety of biological molecules.

Monoclonal hypothesis A hypothesis of how *atherosclerotic plaques* develop. It states that these plaques are benign tumors, each of which is formed by progeny of a single cell that has lost control of its growth and thus proliferates abnormally in the arterial linings.

Monovalent cation tracers Radioactive tracers that lodge in the *heart* in proportion to blood flow and are used to detect portions of the heart that are deprived of blood as a result of blockage of the *coronary arteries.*

Multiple risk factor intervention trial A prospective *clinical trial* now being conducted by the National Heart, Lung, and Blood Institute. Its goal is to determine whether encouraging men to reduce three *risk factors* for heart disease (cigarette smoking, *hypertension,* and high concentrations of serum *cholesterol*) will reduce their incidence of heart disease.

Myocardium *Heart* muscle.

National exercise and heart disease project A prospective *clinical trial* designed to determine whether exercise will extend the life-spans of *heart attack* patients.

Nitroglycerin A drug used to treat *angina pectoris.* It is also being tested as a potential therapy for limiting *infarct* size in *heart attack* victims.

Noradrenalin See *norepinephrine.*

Norepinephrine A *catecholamine* that is a powerful *vasoconstrictor* and that increases *blood pressure.*

Pacemaker, artificial An electrical device used to regulate the beating of the *heart* when the *intrinsic pacemaker* is not working properly.

Pacemaker, intrinsic *Heart* cells in the *sinoatrial node* that set the rhythm of heartbeats by sending out periodic electrical signals that stimulate the *atria,* and then the *ventricles,* to contract.

Placebo An inert substance used as a control in testing the efficacy of drugs or medical procedures.

Platelets Small disc-like bodies in the blood that play an important role in *blood clotting.*

Practolol A *β-blocking agent* being tested for antiarrhythmic activity.

Procaine amide A drug used for treating *cardiac arrhythmias.*

Propranolol (Propanolol) A *β-blocking agent.* Currently, it is the only *β*-blocker registered by the Food and Drug Administration for treatment of *cardiac arrhythmias* and *hypertension.*

Prospective studies *Epidemiological* studies in which groups of people are followed for years in order to determine which persons develop particular diseases. For example, the *Framingham Study* is a prospective study.

Prostacyclin A highly unstable *prostaglandin* (designated PGI$_2$) that contains a ring structure and that prevents or reverses *platelet* aggregation.

Prostaglandins Hormone-like regulatory compounds that affect most body cells and tissues.

Pump failure A condition that occurs when the *heart* is so severely damaged by a *heart attack* that it cannot pump well enough to maintain the *blood pressure*. As the pressure falls, the heart muscle receives progressively less oxygen and may eventually stop pumping.

Quinidine A drug used to treat *cardiac arrhythmias*.

Rabbit aorta contracting substance A substance identified by its contracting effect on rabbit aortas. It may be identical to *thromboxane* A$_2$.

Radionuclide tracers A group of radioactive substances. Some are used to detect defects in blood flow to damaged areas of the *heart*.

Receptors Molecules on the surfaces of cells that bind specific substances, such as hormones, and mediate the physiological effects of those substances.

Renin An *enzyme* produced by the kidney that helps to regulate *blood pressure* by catalyzing the production of *angiotensin*.

Response-to-injury hypothesis A hypothesis of how *atherosclerotic plaques* develop. It proposes that chronic damage to the *arteries* initiates plaque development.

Retrospective studies *Epidemiological* studies in which groups of people are examined at a particular time, and then their backgrounds and histories are assessed to see what may have predisposed them to develop certain diseases or conditions.

Rheumatic heart disease A disease affecting the *heart valves* and muscle. It usually afflicts children between the ages of 5 and 15 and is the result of infection by certain streptococcal bacteria.

Risk factors Conditions that, on the basis of *epidemiological* studies, predispose people to develop certain diseases or disorders.

For example, well-known risk factors for heart disease are cigarette smoking, *hypertension,* and high concentrations of serum *cholesterol.*

Saralasin A drug that, at low doses, antagonizes the action of *angiotensin* and thereby lowers *blood pressure.*

Saturated fat A fat molecule that has only single bonds between its carbon atoms. Saturated fats, such as those in butter, are solids at room temperature.

Scintillation camera A camera that detects radioactivity. It is used to produce images of the *heart* after the organ has been labeled with a radioactive substance.

Sinoatrial node A small strip of *heart* tissue located in the right *atrium* near the spot where the blood enters the heart from the *veins.* The sinoatrial node is the heart's *intrinsic pacemaker.*

Stress An external event or environment that elicits a particular set of physiological responses (the "fight, flight, or fright" reaction) in an individual; alternatively, the physiological and psychological changes produced in a person responding to the stimulus or environment.

Stress electrocardiogram An *electrocardiogram* obtained when a person's *heart* is stressed, usually by exercise such as walking a treadmill. Stress electrocardiograms are used to detect disturbances in the heartbeat that may not be apparent when the patient is at rest.

Stroke Damage to a portion of the brain that results when *arteries* in the brain are blocked by *blood clots* or *atherosclerotic plaques* or when an artery ruptures.

Sudden death Death that occurs within a few minutes because the *heart* stops beating. Often sudden death is caused by *ventricular fibrillation.*

Sympathetic nervous system The branch of the *autonomic nervous system* that helps the organism respond to *stress.*

Systole The part of the *heart's* cycle in which the heart contracts. Systole alternates with *diastole.*

Tachycardia An abnormally fast heartbeat.

Thrombin A natural promotor of *blood clotting.*

Thrombosis A *heart attack* caused by blockage of one or more *coronary arteries* by a kind of *blood clot.*

Thromboxane A close chemical relative of the *prostaglandins*. One particular thromboxane (called TXA_2) causes blood *platelets* to clump and *arteries* to constrict.

Tocainide An experimental drug for controlling *arrhythmias*.

Tomography The technique of making radiographs of plane sections of the body to focus on detail in a predetermined plane.

Transmission tomography *Computerized tomography* that relies on the transmission of x-rays through the body to produce two-dimensional, cross-sectional images of body organs.

Triglycerides Compounds composed of glycerol and fatty acids.

Type A personality A behavior pattern characterized by excessive time-urgency, impatience, competitiveness, aggression, and hostility. It has been linked with an increased risk of *heart attack*.

Type B personality A behavior pattern lacking the type A characteristics. Individuals with this personality may be at lower risk of having a *heart attack*.

Ultrasound imaging Images made when sound with frequencies greater than 20,000 hertz is beamed at an organ. For example, *heart* structures and movements can be detected and *congenital* heart *defects*, heart enlargement, and defects in *heart valves* can be diagnosed by ultrasound imaging.

Unsaturated fat Fat molecules that contain at least one double bond linking their carbon atoms. Unsaturated fats, such as corn oil, are liquids at room temperature.

Unstable angina pectoris *Angina pectoris* that is of recent onset either at rest or on exertion, or angina pectoris that had previously occurred in predictable circumstances (such as after climbing two flights of stairs) and that suddenly begins to occur under different circumstances (such as after climbing one flight of stairs).

Vasoconstrictor An agent that brings about the constriction of any blood vessel, but especially the *arterioles*.

Vasodilation The dilation of any blood vessel.

Vein A vessel that carries blood to the *heart* from the lungs and other tissues of the body.

Ventricles The two lower chambers of the *heart*. These muscular chambers do most of the work of pumping the blood to the rest of the body.

Ventricular fibrillation   Very rapid, uncoordinated contractions of the *ventricles* of the *heart* resulting in loss of synchronization between heartbeat and pulse beat.

Ventricular premature beats   Abnormal heartbeats that occur when the *ventricles* contract earlier in the cardiac cycle than they should. They are considered dangerous because they may result in *ventricular fibrillation* and *sudden death*.

Very-low-density lipoproteins (VLDL)   A class of *lipoproteins* that carry *cholesterol* in the blood.

Vesicles   Small membranous cavities or sacs in cells.

Wolff-Parkinson-White syndrome   A syndrome in which afflicted people have one or more abnormal pathways, in addition to the normal one, for conducting contraction impulses from the *atria* to the *ventricles*. They may suffer attacks of *tachycardia*.

Selected Readings

Epidemiology

1. H. BLACKBURN, "Progress in the Epidemiology and Prevention of Coronary Heart Disease," in *Progress in Cardiology*, P. N. Yu and J. F. Goodwin, eds. Lea and Febiger, Philadelphia, 1974, p. 1.
2. P. MEIER, "Statistics and Medical Experimentation." *Biometrics, 31*, 511 (1975).
3. L. W. SHAW AND T. C. CHALMERS, "Ethics in Cooperative Clinical Trials." *Annals of the New York Academy of Sciences, 196*, 487 (1970).
4. L. WERKÖ, "Risk Factors and Coronary Heart Disease – Facts or Fancy?" *American Heart Journal, 91*, 87 (1976).

Life-Styles and Heart Disease

1. S. M. FOX III, J. P. NAUGHTON, AND W. L. HASKELL, "Physical Activity and the Prevention of Coronary Heart Disease." *Annals of Clinical Research, 3*, 404 (1971).
2. M. FRIEDMAN AND R. H. ROSEMAN, *Type A Behavior and Your Heart.* Alfred A. Knopf, New York, 1974.
3. D. C. GLASS, "Stress, Behavior Patterns, and Coronary Disease." *American Scientist, 65*, 177 (1977).
4. J. N. MORRIS, "Primary Prevention of Heart Attack." *Bulletin of the New York Academy of Medicine, 51*, 62 (1975).
5. A. P. SHAPIRO, G. E. SCHWARTZ, D.C.E. FERGUSON, D. P. REDMOND, AND S. M. WEISS, "Behavioral Methods in the Treatment of Hypertension: A Review of Their Clinical Status." *Annals of Internal Medicine, 86*, 626 (1977).

Etiology

1. E. H. AHRENS, "The Management of Hyperlipidemia: Whether, Rather Than How." *Annals of Internal Medicine, 85*, 87 (1976).
2. E. P. BENDITT, "The Origin of Atherosclerosis." *Scientific American, 236*, 74 (February 1977).
3. M. S. BROWN AND J. L. GOLDSTEIN, "Receptor-Mediated Control of Cholesterol Metabolism." *Science, 191*, 150 (1976).

4. J. D. DAVIS, J. H. LARAGH, AND A. SELWYN, *Hypertension: Mechanisms, Diagnosis, and Management.* HP Publishing Co., New York, 1977. (This book is based on a lengthy series of articles that appeared in *Hospital Practice,* beginning in January 1974.)

5. D. S. FREDERICKSON, J. L. GOLDSTEIN, AND M. S. BROWN, "Familial Hyperlipoproteinemias," in *The Metabolic Basis of Inherited Disease, 4th ed.,* J. B. Wyngaarden and D. S. Frederickson, eds. McGraw-Hill Book Co., New York, 1977.

6. R. ROSS AND J. A. GLOMSET, "The Pathogenesis of Atherosclerosis, Part I." *New England Journal of Medicine, 295,* 369 (1976); "Part II," *ibid.,* p. 420.

7. J. P. WILSON, M. DYE, AND R. CHANCELLOR, *Hypertension Handbook: A Guide for the Patient,* published with the support of a Tennessee Mid-South Regional Medical Program Grant, and available from the office of Dr. John A. Oates, Vanderbilt University Hospital, Nashville, Tennessee. There is a charge of $3.00 for the handbook plus $1.00 for postage and handling.

8. R. W. WISSLER AND D. VESSELINOVITCH, "Studies of Regression of Advanced Atherosclerosis in Experimental Animals and Man." *Annals of the New York Academy of Sciences, 275,* 363 (1976).

Diagnosis and Treatment

1. G. AHUMADA, R. ROBERTS, AND B. E. SOBEL, "Evaluation of Myocardial Infarct with Enzymatic Indices." *Progress in Cardiovascular Disease, 18,* 405 (1976).

2. L. A. COBB, R. S. BAUM, H. ALVAREZ III, AND W. A. SCHAFFER, "Resuscitation from Out-of-Hospital Ventricular Fibrillation." Supplement III to *Circulation, 51* and *52,* III-223 (1975).

3. N. FORTUIN, "Echocardiography: What It Can Do Now." *Hospital Practice, 73* (November 1975).

4. G. GERSTENBLITH, E. G. LAKATTA, AND M. L. WEISFELDT, "Changes in Myocardial Function and Exercise Response." *Progress in Cardiovascular Diseases, 19,* 1 (1976).

5. "Improvement in Prognosis of Myocardial Infarction by Long-Term Beta-Adrenoreceptor Blockade Using Practolol: A Multicentre International Study." *British Medical Journal, 3,* 735 (1975).

6. M. V. JELINEK AND B. LOWN, "Exercise Stress Testing for Exposure of Cardiac Arrhythmia." *Progress in Cardiovascular Disease, 16,* 497 (1974).

7. P. K. MAROKO, J. K. KJEKSHUS, B. E. SOBEL, T. WATANABE, J. W. COVELL, J. ROSS, JR., AND E. BRAUNWALD, "Factors Influencing Infarct Size Following Experimental Coronary Artery Occlusions." *Circulation, 43,* 67 (1971).

8. B. PITT AND H. W. STRAUSS, "Myocardial Imaging in the Noninvasive Evaluation of Patients with Suspected Ischemic Heart Disease." *American Journal of Cardiology, 37,* 797 (1976).

9. R. S. Ross, "The Problem of Ischemic Heart Disease: Current Approaches and Implications for Curriculum Design." *Johns Hopkins Medical Journal, 138,* 217 (1976).

10. E. H. WOOD, "New Horizons for Study of the Cardiopulmonary and Circulatory Systems." *Chest, 69,* 394 (1976).

Index

ACS, *see* American Cancer Society
AHA, *see* American Heart Association
AMIS, *see* Aspirin Myocardial Infarction Study
ATP, *see* adenosine triphosphate
Achuff, Stephen, 158
adenosine triphosphate, heart activity, 140
adrenalin, *see* epinephrine
adrenocorticotrophic hormone, 40
Ahrens, Edward, 63, 64, 65, 68
Albany Medical College, 75, 85
Alderman, E. L., 159
aldosterone, 102–105, 110
alprenolol, 147, 148
Amer, M. Samir, 109
American Cancer Society, 14, 15, 18
American Gastroenterological Association, 26
American Heart Association, x, 3, 25, 114
Anderson, Richard, 79
Anderson, Robert, 152
angina pectoris, 8, 96
  aspirin research, 99
  atherosclerotic plaques, 61
  clinical trials, 27, 163, 164
  coronary bypass surgery, 157–160, 164
  coronary bypass surgery and effects of drugs, 27
  drug treatment, 162
  heart damage, 122
  NHLBI studies, 27
  nitroglycerin treatment, 136
  scintillation camera images, 123

  unstable, 163–164
  Veterans Administration studies, 27, 162
angiograms, *see* coronary angiograms
angiotensin, 112
  blood–brain relationship, 108
  blood pressure regulation, 46, 102, 107
  nervous system relationship, 102
  norepinephrine release, 102
  structures, 103
  synthesis, 106
  vasoconstriction, 104
angiotensinogen, 102, 103
animal experiments, 20
  arteries, 71
  atherosclerosis studies, 69, 73, 84, 85
  blood pressure, 108
  drug–blood pressure relationship, 112
  enzymes, 137
  heart attacks, 134
  hypertension–blood pressure studies, 109
  stress, 43, 109
  sympathetic nervous system, 109
antiarrhythmic drugs, 148, 149, 169
aprindine, 148–149
arachidonic acid, 92, 96, 98
Armstrong, Mark, 85
arrhythmias, *see* cardiac arrhythmias
arterial aneurysm, ix
arterial endothelium, 69–71, 73, 74

This book was set in Century
Expanded and Gill Sans Bold.
It was printed and bound by Waverly
Press, Baltimore, Maryland.

Book design by Ellen Kahan
Production by Anne Holdsworth
Editorial coordination by Kathryn Wolff